# Perceptions of a Pandemic

*Perceptions of a Pandemic* is a thorough and systematic exploration, rooted in data, of the events during the first pandemic of the social media era. This book highlights how the internet and social media have changed how a pandemic can be managed and how essential they have become in our daily lives during crises.

—*Pasi Moisio*, **Research Professor, National Institute for Health and Welfare, Finland**

*Perceptions of a Pandemic* provides a unique look at how the COVID-19 pandemic unfolded during its early months. The wide-ranging analyses offer us insights into how two cultures handled the pandemic, and the results provide guidance for how to manage health emergencies. The authors manage to say something new about the pandemic, which is hard to do at this point. *Perceptions of a Pandemic* is a must read for scholars, policy makers, and anyone who is interested in being better prepared for coping with or managing crises.

—*Matthew Costello*, **Associate Professor, Clemson University, USA**

This work illustrates the enduring value of cross-national comparative sociological analysis. It highlights the similarities and differences between the United States and Finland and then leverages these to examine how the structural features of each country are related to their response to a common exogenous shock: the COVID-19 pandemic. This approach makes a valuable contribution to the literature that goes beyond a single historical event to demonstrate the importance of comparative work for a wide range of topics.

—*James Witte*, **Professor, George Mason University, USA**

# Perceptions of a Pandemic: A Cross-Continental Comparison of Citizen Perceptions, Attitudes, and Behaviors During COVID-19

EDITED BY

**JAMES HAWDON**
*Virginia Tech, USA*

**DONNA SEDGWICK**
*Virginia Tech, USA*

**C. COZETTE COMER**
*Virginia Tech, USA*

AND

**PEKKA RÄSÄNEN**
*University of Turku, Finland*

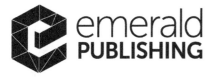

United Kingdom – North America – Japan – India – Malaysia – China

Emerald Publishing Limited
Emerald Publishing, Floor 5, Northspring, 21-23 Wellington Street, Leeds LS1 4DL.

First edition 2025

Editorial matter and selection © 2025 James Hawdon, Donna Sedgwick, C. Cozette Comer, and Pekka Räsänen.
Individual chapters © 2025 The authors.
Published under exclusive licence by Emerald Publishing Limited.

**Reprints and permissions service**
Contact: www.copyright.com

No part of this book may be reproduced, stored in a retrieval system, transmitted in any form or by any means electronic, mechanical, photocopying, recording or otherwise without either the prior written permission of the publisher or a licence permitting restricted copying issued in the UK by The Copyright Licensing Agency and in the USA by The Copyright Clearance Center. Any opinions expressed in the chapters are those of the authors. Whilst Emerald makes every effort to ensure the quality and accuracy of its content, Emerald makes no representation implied or otherwise, as to the chapters' suitability and application and disclaims any warranties, express or implied, to their use.

**British Library Cataloguing in Publication Data**
A catalogue record for this book is available from the British Library

ISBN: 978-1-83608-625-3 (Print)
ISBN: 978-1-83608-624-6 (Online)
ISBN: 978-1-83608-626-0 (Epub)

Printed and bound by CPI Group (UK) Ltd, Croydon, CR0 4YY

INVESTOR IN PEOPLE

*We dedicate this book to the over 7 million people who lost their lives to COVID-19, their families, and their loved ones.*

# Contents

| | |
|---|---|
| List of Figures and Tables | *ix* |
| About the Editors | *xi* |
| About the Contributors | *xiii* |
| Acknowledgments | *xv* |

### Section 1
### Understanding COVID-19: Behaviors, Perceptions, and Solutions

**Chapter 1  Perceptions of a Pandemic: The Impact of COVID-19 on American and Finnish Societies**
*James Hawdon, Donna Sedgwick, C. Cozette Comer and Pekka Räsänen*  3

**Chapter 2  Planned Behavioral Changes to Mitigate COVID-19's Effects**
*James Hawdon*  15

**Chapter 3  Which Factors Contributed to the COVID-19 Outbreak to Become a Global Pandemic?**
*Pekka Räsänen and Aki Koivula*  29

**Chapter 4  Public Priorities During a Pandemic: Cross-national Comparisons**
*C. Cozette Comer*  49

### Section 2
### Media as a Complicating Factor

**Chapter 5  Trust in Experts According to Media Consumption and Government Satisfaction in the United States and Finland**
*Aki Koivula, Eetu Marttila and Pekka Räsänen*  65

*viii*    *Contents*

**Chapter 6    COVID-19 and the Flames of Hate**
*James Hawdon*                                                                      *85*

**Section 3**
**COVID-19 and the Public: Well-being, Compliance,**
**and Health Outcomes**

**Chapter 7    Coping, Well-being, and COVID-19**
*Donna Sedgwick*                                                                    *107*

**Chapter 8    Compliance with Protective Health Behaviors**
**During COVID-19: Variations Over Time and by Country**
*Donna Sedgwick*                                                                    *125*

**Chapter 9    The Pandemic's Effects in Finland and the**
**United States: The Long-term Consequences of Early**
**Perceptions and Behaviors**
*James Hawdon and Donna Sedgwick*                                                    *143*

**Section 4**
**A Look Ahead**

**Chapter 10    A Look Ahead: How to Better Handle the Next**
**Pandemic and Other Crises**
*James Hawdon, Donna Sedgwick, C. Cozette Comer and*
*Pekka Räsänen*                                                                      *171*

Methodological Appendix                                                             *183*

Index                                                                               *199*

# List of Figures and Tables

## Figures

| | | |
|---|---|---|
| Fig. 2.1. | New COVID-19 Cases Per Million Residents. | 19 |
| Fig. 2.2. | New COVID-19 Deaths Per Million Residents. | 20 |
| Fig. 2.3. | Percent Residents Expressing Varying Levels of Concern About the Pandemic. | 20 |
| Fig. 2.4. | Percent Residents Expressing Likelihood of Engaging in Various Behaviors. | 21 |
| Fig. 2.5. | Percent Residents Reporting Plans to Change None of the Listed Behaviors and Percent Planning to Change All 11 Listed Behaviors by Country. | 26 |
| Fig. 3.1. | Citizen Perceptions of the Causes of Pandemic in Spring and Autumn 2020, Shares of Agreement (%) and Margins of Error (95% Confidence Level). | 37 |
| Fig. 3.2. | Predicted Perceptions of the Causes of Pandemic in Spring (Round 1) and Autumn (Round 2) by Political Preference. Probabilities of Agreement with Margins of Errors. | 41 |
| Fig. 4.1. | Percent of Respondents Willing to Increase National Debt to Address COVID-19. | 51 |
| Fig. 4.2. | Percent of Respondents Wanting to Reduce, Maintain, or Increase Each Spending Category by Country. | 52 |
| Fig. 5.1. | Trust in Experts' Capability to Solve COVID-19 Crisis, Satisfaction with Government Response to COVID-19 Crisis, and Daily Media Consumption Patterns in Finland and the United States in the T1 and T2 (Percentages). | 75 |
| Fig. 5.2. | Trust in Experts in Finland and the United States According to Satisfaction with Government Response to COVID-19 Crisis. | 77 |
| Fig. 5.3. | The Effect of Daily Media Consumption Patterns on Trust in Experts. | 78 |
| Fig. 6.1. | Exposure to Online Hate in Finland and the United States: 2020. | 92 |
| Fig. 6.2. | Exposure to Online Hate in Finland and the United States Among Young: 2013 and 2020. | 93 |

## x   List of Figures and Tables

| | | |
|---|---|---|
| Fig. 6.3. | Changes in Exposure to Online Hate Between April and November 2020. | 94 |
| Fig. 7.1. | Factors That Affect Maladaptive Coping: The United States and Finland. | 111 |
| Fig. 7.2. | Factors That Affect Active/Expressive and Planning Coping: The United States and Finland. | 113 |
| Fig. 7.3. | Factors That Affect Positive Reframing Coping: The United States and Finland. | 114 |
| Fig. 7.4. | Factors That Affect Religious Coping: The United States and Finland. | 115 |
| Fig. 7.5. | Predictors of Change in Life Satisfaction in November 2020: The United States and Finland. | 119 |
| Fig. 9.1. | Percent of Respondents Who Wore a Mask in Public During COVID-19. | 150 |

## Tables

| | | |
|---|---|---|
| Table 3.1. | Predicted Perceptions of the Causes of Pandemic in the United States. | 39 |
| Table 3.2. | Predicted Perceptions of the Causes of Pandemic in Finland. | 40 |
| Table AI. | Predicted Perceptions of the Causes of Pandemic in the United States and Finland. | 47 |
| Table 4.1. | Factors Predicting Public Spending Priorities in Finland and the United States: Welfare Spending, Development Spending, and Security Spending. | 54 |
| Table 5.1. | Descriptive Statistics. | 73 |
| Table 5.2. | Trust in Experts According to Satisfaction with Government, Media Consumption Patterns, and Control Variables. | 76 |
| Table 6.1. | Logistic Regression of Exposure to Online Hate in Finland and the United States. | 95 |
| Table 7.1. | Summary of the Significant Predictors with Their Direction for Coping Strategies: Finland and the United States. | 116 |
| Table 8.1. | Mean Compliance and Difference with Mask Wearing in Finland and the United States, April 2020 and November 2020. | 127 |
| Table 8.2. | Factors That Affect Compliance with Mask Wearing April 2020 and November 2020. | 131 |
| Table 8.3. | Factors That Affect Vaccine Intention, November 2020. | 136 |
| Table 9.1. | Logistic Regression of Vaccination Status in the United States and Finland. | 155 |
| Table 9.2. | Regression of Collaborative Relationship with the State in the United States and Finland. | 158 |

# About the Editors

**James Hawdon** is a Professor of Sociology and Director of the Center for Peace Studies and Violence Prevention at Virginia Tech. His research focuses on how communities influence crime, political participation, and responses to tragedies. His recent research has focused on online communities and how they affect political polarization, online hate, and cybercrime. With eight authored or edited books, over 120 academic journal articles and chapters, and dozens of technical reports, he has published extensively in the areas of online extremism, criminology, the sociology of policing, and the sociology of drugs.

**Donna Sedgwick**, PhD, is an Associate Professor in the Department of Sociology at Virginia Tech. Her scholarship includes examining interorganizational relationships between public and nonprofit organizations, and she also investigates how institutional pressures and logics shape organizational and employee behaviors. She has published papers that address these issues on important topics such as early childhood education, policing, affordable housing, and the impact of the COVID-19 pandemic.

**C. Cozette Comer** is the Assistant Director of Evidence Synthesis Services at the University Libraries at Virginia Tech. She specializes in evidence synthesis review methodologies (e.g., systematic reviews and meta-analyses), comprehensive search design, formal critical appraisal of research, and large review management. She is currently a part-time PhD student in Public Administration and Public Affairs, and holds a MS in Sociology from Virginia Tech. Her primary research interests concern the role of evidence in policy and government decision-making.

**Pekka Räsänen**, PhD, is Professor of Economic Sociology at the University Turku, Finland. His research interests are in the sociology of consumption, social inequalities, and the use of information and communication technologies. He has published more than 70 articles in international refereed journals and over 200 other publications. His latest international monograph dealt with exposure to harmful online content among young adults (*Online Hate and Harmful Content – Cross-National Perspectives*, Routledge, 2017).

# About the Contributors

**Aki Koivula** holds the title of docent in Economic Sociology and works as a Senior Researcher at the University of Turku. His research expertise lies in survey research methods, the reciprocal relationship between citizens and public institutions, and people's participation and interaction in digital environments.

**Eetu Marttila** is a Doctoral Researcher in Economic Sociology at the University of Turku. His research explores the effects of social media on individuals' well-being and behavior, specifically in the context of excessive use.

# Acknowledgments

We would like to thank the University of Turku, Economic Sociology Unit, for generously supporting our data collection efforts. We also thank Emmi Lehtinen for providing valuable help with the initial coding of the data. We also thank the University Libraries at Virginia Tech and the Center for Peace Studies and Violence Prevention for hosting our writers' workshop. We also thank our anonymous reviewers. Finally, we thank our families for their love and continued support.

Section 1

# Understanding COVID-19: Behaviors, Perceptions, and Solutions

Chapter 1

# Perceptions of a Pandemic: The Impact of COVID-19 on American and Finnish Societies

*James Hawdon[a], Donna Sedgwick[a], C. Cozette Comer[a] and Pekka Räsänen[b]*

[a] *Virginia Tech, USA*
[b] *University of Turku, Finland*

## Abstract

The introduction provides an overview of the book and explains what the book adds to the literature on the COVID-19 pandemic. It describes the cross-national surveys used for the analyses and the types of questions that are asked in the book. We also explain why the United States and Finland were selected as our comparative cases and detail how this comparison provides a valuable lens for understanding the pandemic. Both nations are liberal democracies with highly developed economies, both score high in terms of compliance with the rule of law, both constitutionally guarantee freedom of speech and a free press, and both share similar cultural factors such has high levels of secularism, self-expression, happiness, social capital, and individualism. Both nations also have well-developed healthcare systems, and both nations were in similar economic positions that positioned them well to pivot to an online economy. Despite these similarities, the nations differ dramatically in size and position in the world system. They also differ with respect to their welfare systems and political systems. Finns also trust their government more than Americans trust theirs, and Finns have historically supported an interventionist state while Americans have always been anti-statism. Finally, another cross-national difference that likely influenced how people perceived the pandemic is the relative levels of security in each nation. With its more generous welfare system, Finns would be more

---

Perceptions of a Pandemic: A Cross-Continental Comparison of Citizen Perceptions, Attitudes, and Behaviors During COVID-19, 3–14

Copyright © 2025 by James Hawdon, Donna Sedgwick, C. Cozette Comer and Pekka Räsänen

Published under exclusive licence by Emerald Publishing Limited

doi:10.1108/978-1-83608-624-620241001

# 4 *James Hawdon et al.*

confident about successfully navigating the pandemic than would Americans. The chapter ends with a brief description of how each substantive chapter is outlined.

*Keywords*: Finland; United States; COVID-19; cross-national comparisons; survey data

## Introduction

The first cases of severe acute respiratory syndrome coronavirus 2 (SARS-CoV-2), or COVID-19 as it came to be called, were reported in Wuhan, China, in December 2019. Shortly thereafter, China began to report thousands of new cases. Despite efforts to contain the virus, including shutting down travel into and out of the city of Wuhan, other countries began reporting cases (Taylor, 2021). Japan, South Korea, Thailand, and the United States reported cases by late January 2020, and the World Health Organization (WHO) declared a "public health emergency of international concern" on January 30, 2020.

From there, the situation quickly grew worse as the virus's deadly seriousness became fully understood. News of COVID-19 deaths outside of China, including the Philippines in early February and France in mid-February, demonstrated the virus had spread across the globe. Then truly horrific scenes from areas hit particularly hard, such as in the Lombardy region of northern Italy, proved sobering. Even well-equipped hospitals systems were struggling to care for a seemingly endless supply of very sick patients, and the forecasted future became increasingly grim. Images of exhausted healthcare workers donning full personal protective equipment (PPE) caring for patients on respirators started to dominate the news while the virus continued its deadly spread to Iran, Brazil, India, South Africa, Israel; indeed, it was spreading throughout Europe, Asia, Africa, Oceana, and the Americas. On March 11, 2020, the WHO identified COVID-19 as a pandemic (WHO, 2020), and by April 1, 2020, the pandemic had infected more than one million people in 171 countries and had killed at least 51,000 (Taylor, 2021).

There have of course been prior global health crises. The Influenza Pandemic of 1918 or "Spanish Flu" infected approximately one-third of the world's population and killed approximately 50 million people (Center for Disease Control (CDC), 2018).[1] The 1968 $H_3N_2$ pandemic killed over 1 million worldwide (Center for Disease Control (CDC), 2019). SARS-CoV-1 ravaged south China between November 2002 and July 2003, and over 8,000 people became sick and more than 700 died before the WHO declared the outbreak as being over (Center for Disease Control (CDC), 2022). MERS-CoV, which was first reported in Saudi Arabia in

---

[1]Some estimates suggest even 100 million died of the 1918 pandemic as numbers were difficult to track given that nations involved in WWI tried to downplay the toll the disease was having on their soldiers and home fronts.

2012, has now spread to people in 27 countries, and over 2.6 million have become ill and nearly 900 have died of MERS since (European Centre for Disease Prevention and Control, 2022). So, humans have dealt with pandemics before, and despite the awful suffering these have caused, the species survived and those who did went on with their lives. This will be the likely outcome of the COVID-19 pandemic as well; however, there is an important difference between the current pandemic and those of our past. The social world is a far smaller place today than it was in 1918, 1969, 2003, and even 2012. As such, our mitigation strategies had far more profound consequences.

As it became obvious that COVID-19 was a deadly and highly contagious disease, healthcare providers and government officials called on citizens to practice health-protective behaviors to quell the pandemic. We were informed of the need to "flatten the curve" to prevent our healthcare systems from being overwhelmed. We were told not only to practice typical preventative behaviors, such as handwashing and covering coughs, but also to adopt behaviors more specific to COVID-19. In many places, these calls for health-protective behaviors included stay-at-home orders, maintaining 6 ft (2 m) social distance from non-family members, and wearing a face covering when in public (Finnish Government, 2020; Sedgwick et al., 2022; Welker et al., 2020). Similar measures were taken in the past as well, but never to the extent that we witnessed in 2020. Our truly global, truly interdependent economy ground to a crawl. Between 2019 and 2020, the world's real GDP fell by 3.6%, the volume of trade declined by over 5%, and foreign direct investment dropped by 42% (Zhang, 2021; also see Oum et al., 2022). This was unquestionably the worst economic downturn since the Great Depression. Moreover, as we were told to stay home and avoid public places, our work behaviors, our leisure behaviors, our religious behaviors, our consuming behaviors, and a variety of other behaviors changed. Indeed, it seemed like everything changed!

While it is undeniable that COVID-19 dramatically affected our behaviors, exactly which behaviors – from teleworking to media consumption to mask wearing and handwashing – changed because of the pandemic? What perceptions and attitudes, such as trust in institutions (e.g., government, universities, and hospitals) and attitudes toward science, patterned these behaviors and any changes that occurred in them? How do these factors relate to opinions of policy, such as how we should be spending money during a pandemic and who (e.g., government, universities, and hospitals) is best suited to get us out of the pandemic? And did any of our changed behaviors or attitudes affect the likelihood of us or our loved ones getting sick? Our research aims to answer these questions by examining survey data collected at two time points during the early stages of the COVID-19 pandemic – March/April and October 2020 – in the United States and Finland. Social science plays a pivotal role in understanding health-related topics, particularly when trying to understand disease spread during global pandemics and the behaviors individuals do – and do not do – when trying to mitigate that spread. In the earliest stages of a pandemic, having citizens comply with health-protective behaviors is critical in slowing the viruses' spread as compliance can provide medical institutions time to develop effective treatment protocols and the scientific community time to develop vaccines and treatment drugs (Bish &

## 6  James Hawdon et al.

Michie, 2010). Thus, understanding the perception, attitudes, and behaviors that pattern compliance is vital for advancing effective policies that are well informed by social science.

## What Can We Add to the Conversation?

There are literally millions of academic books, book chapters, peer-reviewed journal articles, policy briefs, governmental white papers, and journalistic accounts related to COVID-19. A simple search in Google Scholar for "COVID-19" returns over 4.7 million results. It is undoubtedly difficult to say much of anything new on this topic; however, we are confident that our approach allows us to do so. We conducted a series of analyses that address these issues and contribute to the growing body of research aimed at mitigating the effects of the current and future health crises. The focus on how perceptions and behaviors changed *during the early stages of the pandemic* will allow us to capture peoples' initial reactions, attitudes, beliefs, and fears. Moreover, our cross-national approach is relatively unique, even among the 4.7 million other works on the topic.

While existing work on COVID-19 is extremely valuable, our focus affords a broader perspective than the vast majority of these works by detailing how the pandemic differentially unfolded in two countries. As such, our approach has several unique strengths. First, it offers a comparative study about the societal effects of the pandemic between the United States and Finland – two countries with very different social welfare systems and relationships between citizens and government. Second, the study data are unique. The data were collected at three points of time, and the first two waves of data were collected from a panel of respondents. This design allows for analyses of the early and later responses to the pandemic. Third, the survey questions cover a wide-range of topics connected to the pandemic, including perceptions about well-being and the possible causes and solutions of COVID-19, and behaviors undertaken, such as mask wearing, consumption activities, and exposure to online hate. This range offers a broad understanding of how COVID-19 shaped citizens' lives in both counties. Fourth, this book offers a unique methodological approach of investigating multiple issues connected to a phenomenon using one comparative data set (at two points in time). This allows readers to assess the quality of the information overall (rather than having to assess for each contributed chapter) and delve deeply into the topics and comparisons. Finally, as the pandemic unfolded, it became increasingly politicized as one's willingness to wear masks and be vaccinated became strongly affiliated with political party. Our data capture the perceptions of the pandemic prior to it becoming intensely political. By focusing on early perceptions and how these changed, we capture peoples' initial reactions and perceptions. This focus will not only allow us to consider the possible causes as to how the pandemic differentially unfolded in the two countries but also better inform future policymakers when new health crises emerge. By studying the early reactions to the pandemic, we will be able to highlight the issues and challenges future policymakers will need to consider if they are to successfully avoid the partisanship that has thwarted efforts to combat the COVID-19 pandemic.

## Why Finland and the United States?

Although several books have been published on the many social facets of the COVID-19, to our knowledge, our book is unique in its cross-national focus on two comparable, yet diverging countries. But why, out of the 193 countries on earth, look at the United States and Finland?

First, Finland and the United States have many similarities. They are both liberal democracies with highly developed economies, with the United States having the 12th highest GDP per capita and Finland having the 21st (World Bank, 2021). Both nations score high in terms of compliance with the rule of law and the regulatory quality of a government, with Finland receiving a perfect score of 100 and the United States a score of 81 on a scale from 0 to 100 (Worlddata, 2022). Both nations also constitutionally guarantee freedom of speech and a free press. There are cultural similarities too. For example, both nations score high on the Inglehart–Welzel's secularism and self-expression scales (see Inglehart et al., 2014). In fact, they have nearly identical scores on the self-expression scale, which reflects tolerance of diversity. They also have similar levels of expressed happiness, with over 92% of both Americans and Finns reporting that they are either "quite happy" or "very happy" (Inglehart et al., 2014). Both nations also enjoy among the highest levels of social capital and individualism in the world (see Allik & Realo, 2004).

Finland and the United States also have important similarities with respect to factors that relate to how COVID-19 was handled. For example, both countries have well-developed healthcare systems. Based on the CEOWORLD Magazine's Health Care Index, Finland has the fifth best healthcare system and the United States has the 18th best (World Population Review, 2022). Importantly for handling the COVID-19 crises, Finland has approximately 3.6 hospital beds per 1,000 population and the United States has 2.9 hospital beds per 1,000 population. As such, both nations were reasonably well positioned to cope with the burden COVID-19 placed on their healthcare systems. The nations also were in similar positions with respect to economic factors. Both nations are dominated by the service sector, with 79.1% of American laborers and 78.4% of Finnish laborers working in the service sector (Central Intelligence Agency (CIA), 2022). Moreover, they were both well positioned to pivot to an online economy since both are among the world's leading nations in term of internet penetration with over 90% of the population having internet access (International Telecommunication Union (ITU), 2021).

Second, while the two nations have numerous similarities that make them comparable in many ways, they also have important differences that make the comparison interesting and informative. First and foremost, the two nations differ dramatically with respect to their size and position in the world system. Finland is a small nation of approximately 5.6 million people. The United States is nearly 60 times larger at 333.3 million people. The United States is the third most populist nation while Finland is the 118th. Moreover, while both nations are considered "core" nations (Babones, 2005; Chase-Dunn et al., 2000), the United States is the most dominant nation in the world system.

**8** *James Hawdon et al.*

Next, the two nations have very different welfare systems. Finland is a classic Nordic welfare state (e.g., Esping-Andersen, 1990; Räsänen, 2006) where the state provides its citizens with universal coverage of old age pensions, sickness insurance, occupational injury insurance, child allowance, and parental leave (see Greve, 2007; Lin, 2004). This system has extensive fiscal intervention in the labor market, and the marginal tax rates are high (Alesina & Glaeser, 2006). By comparison, the American welfare model is based on "minimal state interference" (Hass, 2006, p. 69), and the government in the United States becomes involved in welfare provision only when the market, voluntary organizations, and the family fail to provide services (see Gilbert, 2002). As an "enabling state" (Gilbert, 2002), the US state mandates private social welfare expenditures or finance services either directly through contracts or vouchers or indirectly through tax incentives (Gilbert, 2002; Katz, 2002). As a result, the US social safety net is comparatively limited.

A third major difference between the nations that likely influenced the perceptions of the pandemic is the political system. While both are representative democracies, the United States is for all intents and purposes a two-party system while Finland is a multi-party system. In the United States, despite having parties such as the Green Party, the Socialist Party, the Libertarian Party, and Independents, only the Democratic and Republican parties offer viable candidates, especially at the federal level. For example, in the 2020 presidential election, Democrat Joe Biden received approximately 81.3 million votes, Republican Donald Trump received slightly over 74.2 million votes, and Libertarian Jo Jorgensen received a mere 1.9 million votes. In 2016, Green Party candidate Jill Stein received 1.4 million votes and Independent Evan McMullin received 731,911 while Democratic candidate Hillary Clinton received 65.8 million and Republican Donald Trump 62.9 million votes. By contrast, Finland's multi-party system makes it nearly impossible for any one party to win a majority, thereby leading to a coalition government where several political parties are forced to cooperate to form the government. Those parties not in the ruling coalition are "opposition parties." To be recognized as a party, the association must be recorded in the Ministry of Justice's party register. Currently, Finland has 10 Parliamentary parties and 14 non-Parliamentary Parties that are registered but that have not received a seat in the Parliament of Finland nor in the European Parliament.[2]

Next, Finns trust their government far more than Americans trust theirs, which may be related to the party system in each nation that was just discussed. According to Eurostat (2021), Finns express the second highest level of trust in their political system in Europe, following only Switzerland (also see Marien & Hooghe, 2011). By comparison, Americans express far lower levels of trust. Based on recent PEW data, only 17% of Americans say they can trust the government

---

[2]The current Parliamentary parties are Social Democratic Party, the Finns Party, the National Coalition Party, the Centre Party, the Green League, the Left Alliance, the Swedish People's Party, the Christian Democrats, the Movement Now, and the Power Belongs to the People.

in Washington to do what is right at least "most of the time" (PEW Research Center, 2019). Related to levels of trust in the state, Finns have historically supported an interventionist state and a tradition of "statism" (Lin, 2004; Midttun & Witoszek, 2010), but there has always been a strong anti-statism in the United States (Quadagno & Street, 2005).

Finally, like other Nordic states, Finland is characterized by a high degree of equality in terms of disposable income (Lassen & Sorenson, 2002). Conversely, the United States has far higher levels of inequality than typical Scandinavian nations. The two nation's Gini coefficients are telling. The Gini coefficient measures inequality in a nation, with higher numbers representing more inequality. The Gini coefficient for income in the United States is 41.5, which ranks as the 49th most unequal nation in the world. Finland, on the other hand, has one of the lowest levels of inequality in the world. Its Gini coefficient of 27.7 is the 12th lowest (CIA, 2022).

These different institutional arrangements may contribute to both cross-national health differences (see Hurrelmann et al., 2011; Pförtner et al., 2019), and these arrangements are likely to influence if citizens comply with state requests made during the pandemic as these factors affect the relationship between the state and their citizens. First and foremost, as mentioned, the two nations differ dramatically with respect to their welfare systems. Finland is a classic Nordic welfare state (e.g., Esping-Andersen, 1990; Räsänen, 2006) where the state provides its citizens with universal coverage of old age pensions, sickness insurance, occupational injury insurance, child allowance, and parental leave (see Greve, 2007; Lin, 2004). This system has extensive fiscal intervention in the labor market, and the marginal tax rates are high (Alesina & Glaeser, 2006). By comparison, the American welfare model is based on "minimal state interference" (Hass, 2006, p. 69), and the government in the United States becomes involved in welfare provision only as a last resort when the market solutions fail to provide services (see Gilbert, 2002).

The differences in welfare systems are notable with respect to the provision of healthcare. Not only are Finns provided with basic universal health coverage, they also have different health literacy rates. In the United States, a National Assessment of Adult Literacy indicated a 12% health literacy rate in May 2019 (Office of the Surgeon General, 2019). Lacking a national curriculum, the extent to which health literacy is taught in schools varies by distract. In contrast, the national school curricula in Finland includes a health literacy component. According to a WHO (2019) news release, "Finnish pupils are … among the best informed about health in Europe." Although no national assessment of health literacy rates among the general population are available, it can be inferred that this universal approach to health literacy training in Finland has led to an overall better rate compared to the concerningly low health literacy rate in the United States.

Another difference between the two nations is with the relative freedom of the press. The two nations both have constitutional protections for free speech and a tradition of a free press, but press in the United States is less free than that found in Finland, at least according to the World Press Freedom Index. According to Reporters Without Boarders, press freedom is defined the ability of journalists

## 10   *James Hawdon et al.*

"to select, produce, and disseminate news in the public interest independent of political, economic, legal, and social interference and in the absence of threats to their physical and mental safety" (Reporters Without Borders, 2022). They create an index that ranges from 0 to 100 based on a quantitative tally of abuses against journalists and a qualitative analysis of the situation in the country. Using this index, Finland scores an 88.42, which is fifth best in the world. By comparison, the United States scores only a 72.74, which ranks 42nd in the world. The freedom of the press is relevant in terms of how the pandemic was perceived and played out in the two countries because a free press is more likely to provide more balanced coverage of controversies surrounding the pandemic and health mandates. A free press is also more likely to instill confidence in the citizenry that they were being adequately informed about the pandemic. Indeed, trust in the news media in Finland is the highest in the world while the United States ranks last among 46 countries included in a recent Reuters Institute Study (Newman, 2022). Given the trust in the media in Finland and the mistrust of the press in the United States, we would predict that the pandemic would become more political and more controversial in the United States than in Finland.

Finally, another cross-national difference that likely influenced how people perceived the pandemic is the relative levels of security in each nation. With its more generous welfare system, we would predict that Finns would be more confident about successfully navigating the pandemic than would Americans. While Finns could confidently rely on their social safety net to mitigate any financial harms caused by the pandemic, Americans were in a far less stable position. Similarly, Finns knew their healthcare costs would be covered should they or a family member become seriously ill with COVID-19, but many Americans had to worry about what a prolonged illness would do not only to their family's health but also its economic well-being.

Because of the similarities and differences between the two nations, Finland and the United States provide powerful comparative cases. They are similar enough in terms of many of their central institutions – their economic, political, media, and healthcare institutions – to allow for comparisons, but they vary enough on important dimensions – their welfare systems, levels of trust in government, and histories of statism – to anticipate differences in how COVID-19 played out in each nation during the earliest stages of the pandemic.

## The Book

There are ten chapters grouped into three general sections: Understanding COVID-19; Behaviors, Perceptions, and Solutions; Media as a Complicating Factor; and Public Priorities: Spending, Well-being, and Compliance. Each of these sections is based primarily on an analysis of survey data collected in April and November 2020. The ninth chapter is based on a similar data set that was collected in November 2023, approximately 6 months after the pandemic was declared to be over. These data are unique. Unlike many other surveys conducted in 2020, our surveys included many of the same people in both the first and second waves. That is, we have a panel of respondents from two countries. The unique longitudinal

*Perceptions of a Pandemic* **11**

data generated from these surveys permit us to assess the effects of COVID-19 within and between individuals and countries. While our third wave of data is a separate sample and not panel data, we gather data that can tap similar concepts that were used in the first two waves of data and then correlate these with health and well-being outcomes related to the pandemic. We include a technical chapter that describes the data in detail. The chapter also includes detailed descriptions of how all the concepts used in the analyses throughout the book are measured. This chapter will also include all the statistical results for all of the analyses conducted throughout the book. By including this information in the appendix, we will be able to present the findings in the content chapters without the distraction of the methodological and statistical details. This approach will allow the casual reader to concentrate on the findings while still providing the necessary information for the scientific community to assess the rigor and quality of the analyses and hopefully reproduce the work.

The second chapter – and first content chapter – provides an analysis of the behaviors people said they planned to change to mitigate the adverse effects of the pandemic. Using the Theory of Planned Behavior as a frame, the chapter looks at differences between what people in Finland and people in the United States said they planned to do and what factors shaped these plans. The third chapter discusses the perceptions of the causes of the pandemic. From wildlife street markets to globalization and travel, comparisons are made between the two nations in how people viewed the pandemic and what they blamed for it. The chapter is framed using various theories of risk perception and work on the risk society. The fourth chapter and final in this section analyzes public priorities during the pandemic. Specifically, the chapter compares the two nations in terms of attitudes toward public spending. Rooted in theories of public administration, the chapter explores who wanted to increase public spending to combat the pandemic, who was reluctant to have the state assume more debt, and factors that helped shape the desire to spend on different institutions.

In the section on complicating factors, Chapter 5 looks at how media consumption influences trust in experts and government satisfaction in the United States and Finland. The chapter provides a test of the idea that greater diversity in news sources provides a more balanced and non-partisan perspective on topics. The sixth chapter looks at exposure to online hate materials during the pandemic using a routine activities theory lens. It is well documented that hate crimes increased during the pandemic, but we investigate if people saw more online hate and if this exposure was patterned by country.

In the final section of the book, we demonstrate why the perceptions people have early in the pandemic matter. Chapter 7 analyzes cross-national differences in coping strategies and if these strategies affected well-being. Chapter 8 investigates citizen compliance with protective health behaviors. Building on previous work and using collaboration theory, we investigate how attitudes about government and other institutions as well as perceptions about the pandemic influence if one wore a mask, washed their hands, maintained social distance, and expressed willingness to be vaccinated. Chapter 9 looks at the factors that predict who became ill with COVID-19. We predict if the respondent or anyone in her or his family

## 12   James Hawdon et al.

got COVID-19 using the various factors discussed and analyzed throughout the book. We demonstrate that perceptions in the early stages of the pandemic do matter, and these can become matters of life and death. The final chapter uses the insights from the previous chapters to offer policy recommendations for managing the next crisis more effectively. We highlight some of the mistakes that were made as well as some of the good decisions that helped us preserve through the pandemic.

The data and theoretical discussions presented in the book provide rich explanations for variations in perceptions, attitudes, and behaviors as well as a cross-national comparison between two countries with different approaches to governance and social welfare.

# References

Alesina, A., & Glaeser, E. L. (2006). Why are welfare states in the US and Europe so different?. *Horizons Stratégiques*, *2*(2), 51–61.

Allik, J., & Realo, A. (2004). Individualism-collectivism and social capital. *Journal of Cross-Cultural Psychology*, *35*(1), 29–49.

Babones, S. (2005). The country-level income structure of the world-economy. *Journal of World-Systems Research*, *11*(1), 29–55.

Bish, A., & Michie, S. (2010). Demographic and attitudinal determinants of protective behaviours during a pandemic: A review. *British Journal of Health Psychology*, *15*(4), 797–824.

Center for Disease Control (CDC). (2018). *History of 1918 flu pandemic*. https://www.cdc.gov/flu/pandemic-resources/1918-commemoration/1918-pandemic-history.htm

Center for Disease Control (CDC). (2019). *1968 pandemic ($H_3N_2$ virus)*. https://www.cdc.gov/flu/pandemic-resources/1968-pandemic.html#:~:text=It%20was%20first%20noted%20in,a%20seasonal%20influenza%20A%20virus

Center for Disease Control (CDC). (2022). *Severe acute respiratory syndrome (SARS)*. https://www.cdc.gov/sars/about/faq.html

Central Intelligence Agency (CIA). (2022). *CIA world factbook*. https://www.cia.gov/the-world-factbook/

Chase-Dunn, C., Kawano, Y., & Brewer, B. D. (2000). Trade globalization since 1795: Waves of integration in the world-system. *American Sociological Review*, *65*(1), 77–95.

Esping-Andersen, G. (1990). *The three worlds of welfare capitalism*. Princeton University Press.

European Centre for Disease Prevention and Control. (2022). *MERS-CoV worldwide overview*. https://www.ecdc.europa.eu/en/middle-east-respiratory-syndrome-coronavirus-mers-cov-situation-update

Eurostat. (2021). Average rating of trust by domain, sex, age and educational attainment level. *Statistics* | Eurostat (europa.eu).

Finnish Government. (2020). *Information and advice on the coronavirus*. https://valtioneuvosto.fi/en/information-on-coronavirus

Gilbert, N. (2002). *Transformation of the welfare state: The silent surrender of public responsibility*. Oxford University Press.

Greve, B. (2007). What characterise the Nordic welfare state model. *Journal of Social Sciences*, *3*(2), 43–51.

Hass, J. (2006). *Economic sociology: An introduction*. Routledge.

## Perceptions of a Pandemic    13

Hurrelmann, K., Rathmann, K., & Richter, M. (2011). Health inequalities and welfare state regimes. A research note. *Journal of Public Health, 19*(1), 3–13.

Inglehart, R., Haerpfer, C., Moreno, A., Welzel, C., Kizilova, K., Diez-Medrano, J., Lagos, M., Norris, P., Ponarin, E., & Puranen, B. (Eds.). (2014). *World values survey: Round five – Country-pooled datafile version*. JD Systems Institute. www.worldvaluessurvey.org/WVSDocumentationWV5.jsp

International Telecommunication Union (ITU). (2021). *World telecommunication/ICT indicators database* https://www.itu.int/en/ITU-D/Statistics/Pages/publications/wtid.aspx.

Katz, M. B. (2002). *The price of citizenship: Redefining the American welfare state*. Macmillan.

Lassen, D. D., & Sorenson, P. B. (2002). *The challenge of globalization to taxation in the Nordic countries: A report prepared for the Nordic Council of Ministers*. Economic Policy and Research Unit, Institute of Economics, University of Copenhagen, Copenhagen.

Lin, K. (2004). Sectors, agents and rationale: A study of the Scandinavian welfare states with special reference to the welfare society model. *Acta Sociologica, 47*(2), 141–157.

Marien, S., & Hooghe, M. (2011). Does political trust matter? An empirical investigation into the relation between political trust and support for law compliance. *European Journal of Political Research, 50*(2), 267–291.

Midttun, A., & Witoszek, N. (2010). Introduction: The Nordic model-how sustainable or exportable is it? In A. Midttun & N. Witoszek (Eds.), *The Nordic model: Is it sustainable and exportable?* (pp. 5–7). University of Oslo.

Newman, N. (2022). *Overview and key findings of the 2022 digital news report*. Reuters Institute. https://reutersinstitute.politics.ox.ac.uk/digital-news-report/2022/dnr-executive-summary

Office of the Surgeon General. (2019). *Health literacy reports and publications*. https://www.hhs.gov/surgeongeneral/reports-and-publications/health-literacy/index.html

Oum, S., Kates, J., & Wexler, A. (2022). *Economic impact of COVID-19 on PEPFAR countries*. Global Health Policy. https://www.kff.org/global-health-policy/issue-brief/economic-impact-of-covid-19-on-pepfar-countries/#:~:text=The%20toll%20the%20COVID%2D19,downturn%20since%20the%20Great%20Depression

PEW Research Center. (2019). *Public trust in government: 1958–2019*. https://www.pewresearch.org/politics/2019/04/11/public-trust-in-government-1958-2019/

Pförtner, T.-K., Pfaff, H., & Elgar, F. (2019). *The role of welfare state characteristics for health and inequalities in health from a cross-national perspective: A critical research synthesis*. Kölner Zeitschrift für Soziologie und Sozialpsychologie, 71(1), 465–489.

Quadagno, J., & Street, D. (2005). Ideology and public policy: Antistatism in American welfare state transformation. *Journal of Policy History, 17*(1), 52–71.

Räsänen, P. (2006). Consumption disparities in information society: comparing the traditional and digital divides in Finland. *International Journal of Sociology and Social Policy, 26*(1/2), 48–62.

Reporters Without Borders. (2022). *2021 world press freedom index*. https://rsf.org/en/index

Sedgwick, D., Hawdon, J., Räsänen, P., & Koivula, A. (2022). The role of collaboration in complying with COVID-19 health protective behaviors: A cross-national study. *Administration & Society, 54*(1), 29–56.

Taylor, D. B. (2021, March 17). A timeline of the coronavirus pandemic. *The New York Times*. https://www.nytimes.com/article/coronavirus-timeline.html.

Welker, K., Bennett, G., & Clark, D. (2020). CDC recommends people wear cloth masks in public—But Trump says he won't. *NBC News*. https://www.nbcnews.com/news/us-news/u-s-expected-recommend-masks-americans-coronavirus-hotspots-n1175596

World Bank. (2021). *GDP per capita—Current US dollars*. https://data.worldbank.org/indicator/NY.GDP.PCAP.CD?most_recent_value_desc=true

## 14  James Hawdon et al.

World Health Organization. (2019, September 13). *Health literacy counts as academic competence in Finnish schools.* https://www.who.int/europe/news/item/13-09-2019-health-literacy-counts-as-academic-competence-in-finnish-schools

World Health Organization (WHO). (2020, March 11). *Timeline: WHO's COVID-19 response.* https://www.who.int/emergencies/diseases/novel-coronavirus-2019/interactive-timeline.

World Population Review. (2022). *Best healthcare in the world 2022.* https://worldpopulationreview.com/country-rankings/best-healthcare-in-the-world

Worlddata (2022). *Comparison of quality of life worldwide.* https://www.worlddata.info/quality-of-life.php

Zhang, H. (2021). *The impact of COVID-19 on global production.* Centre for Economic Policy Research. https://voxeu.org/article/impact-covid-19-global-production

Chapter 2

# Planned Behavioral Changes to Mitigate COVID-19's Effects

*James Hawdon*

*Virginia Tech, USA*

## Abstract

This chapter analyzes the behaviors people planned to change to mitigate the adverse effects of the pandemic using the Theory of Planned Behavior (TPB) as a frame. The TPB argues that behaviors are largely determined by an individual's intention to engage in the behavior, and behavioral intensions are functions of attitudes, perceived behavioral control, and subjective norms. After reviewing the theoretical perspective, data on respondents' plans to change their leisure activities such as eating in restaurants, buying take-out food or using food delivery services, traveling, gathering in public, and visiting with friends are analyzed. I also look at their planned changes in their use of public transportation, e-commerce, and other online activities. Using factor analysis, behaviors group into two distinct factors: *planned changes to interactions* (e.g., avoiding public gatherings, visit bars and restaurants less often, and visit friends and relatives less often) and *planned changes to consuming behaviors* (e.g., purchasing online services more, ordering take-out food more often). Investigating if planned changes vary across country and respondent attitudes, Finnish respondents were significantly more likely to say they planned to change their *interactions* than were Americans, while Americans were significantly more likely to report they planned to change their *consuming behaviors*. The chapter concludes by considering if people's beliefs about what caused the pandemic explain these observed differences. This was the case in terms of changes to

---

Perceptions of a Pandemic: A Cross-Continental Comparison of Citizen Perceptions, Attitudes, and Behaviors During COVID-19, 15–28

Copyright © 2025 by James Hawdon

Published under exclusive licence by Emerald Publishing Limited

doi:10.1108/978-1-83608-624-620241002

*16    James Hawdon*

*interactions*, but it was not the case for plans to change *consuming behaviors* to mitigate the pandemic's threats.

*Keywords*: Theory of Planned Behavior; Theory of Reasoned Action; mitigation strategies during health crises; consuming behaviors during COVID-19; social interactions during COVID-19

## Introduction

Our world and the normal way of navigating it were abruptly disrupted when SARS-CoV-2, or COVID-19, began infecting people in December 2019. When first reported, something felt different from previous outbreaks of infectious diseases such as SARS-CoV-1 in 2003 and the Middle East respiratory syndrome (or MERS-CoV or MERS) in 2012. This virus seemed to be more infectious, evidenced by thousands of new cases being reported on a near-daily basis despite efforts to contain the virus. By January 2020, cases had spread from China to other countries, including Japan, South Korea, Thailand, and the United States. In about a month, COVID-19 had gone from a disease limited to a city in central China to a WHO-declared "public health emergency of international concern."

It did not take long for COVID-19 to spread across the globe to Europe, Asia, Africa, Oceana, and the Americas nor for its deadly consequences to be seen. Deaths began being recorded in the Philippines, Italy, France, Iran, Brazil, India, South Africa, Israel, the United States, and elsewhere. By April 1, 2020, the pandemic had infected more than one million people and killed at least 51,000 (Taylor, 2021).

As COVID-19 rapidly spread, government officials in several countries called on citizens to practice health protective behaviors such as handwashing, covering coughs, maintaining social distance, avoiding crowds and public transportation, and wearing a mask in public (Finnish Government, 2020; Sedgwick et al., 2022; Welker et al., 2020). With the heightened media coverage and awareness of the threat the virus posed to world health, concern began to spread even faster than the virus. Yet, the virus's spread and concern about it were not uniform across the globe. Official governmental responses to the pandemic also varied cross-nationally. For example, New Zealand immediately shut down all nonessential businesses, banned large social gatherings, and severely restricted international travel (Dyer, 2021). In contrast, Sweden adopted a less restrictive strategy that emphasized individual responsibility, avoided shutting down businesses, and only limited public gatherings of more than 500 people (Giritli Nygren & Olofsson, 2020; Hale et al., 2021). The relative spread of the virus, the concern about it, and the governmental response to it undeniably affected peoples' behaviors. But, what behaviors changed, and what patterned the changes that occurred? While later chapters explore these topics in detail, this chapter focuses on an even more fundamental question: *What behaviors did people **plan to change**?* It is important to first focus on the behavioral changes people said they were likely to make at the

*Planned Behavioral Changes* **17**

beginning of the pandemic because, as explained by the TPB, intended behaviors are related to future behaviors.

## The TPB

Plans to engage in a given behavior should be good predictors of future behaviors, at least according to the Theory of Reasoned Action and its revised version, the TPB. These theories specifically argue that behaviors are largely determined by an individual's intention to engage in the behavior (Ajzen & Fishbein, 1980; Fishbein & Ajzen, 1975). TPB has been applied to several health-related behaviors with moderate success predicting those behaviors (e.g., Ajzen, 1991; Albarracin et al., 2001; Nguyen et al., 1997). Thus, knowing what one plans to do in the future should help us predict their future behaviors. Such predictions are vital for public health officials as they make plans to implement mitigation strategies.

TPB maintains that behavioral intention directly determines behavior, but behavioral intensions are functions of attitudes, perceived behavioral control, and subjective norms. *Attitudes* are the individual's beliefs about a given behavior, and these are determined by the person's assessment that the behavior will produce a specific outcome. According to the theory, an individual's positive evaluation is the belief about the effectiveness of the behavior in reducing the likelihood or risk of negative outcomes, while a negative evaluation is the beliefs about possible adverse consequences that may result from engaging in the behavior. The more positive beliefs relative to negative ones, the greater the likelihood the individual will intend to engage in the behavior. This factor is clearly relevant to performing recommended health-protective behaviors: if someone believes these behaviors will reduce the risk of him or her dying while causing few or no negative consequences, the individual is likely to at least *intend* to engage in those behaviors.

Next, *perceived behavioral control* is an individual's perceptions regarding the ease or difficulty of performing the behavior. Individuals are far more likely to intend to engage in a behavior if they have confidence they can successfully perform the behavior. The extent to which individuals believe they can perform the behavior is a function of the factors actors are aware of that may impede or facilitate the behavior. This additional condition is critical for adopting health-protective behaviors as people are far less likely to engage in behaviors that will require radical changes than they are to engage in behaviors that they can adopt easily.

Finally, the theory specifically includes the social context in which the individual is making decisions about the behavior. This inclusion is critical because behavior is often dependent on the individual's social networks and organizations. TPB defines subjective norms as the individual's perceptions of whether their friends, family, and society expect them to engage in the behavior. Social norms will likely influence one's decisions about performing recommended health-protective behaviors: if people in an actor's social networks strongly believes these behaviors should be practiced, it is likely the people in that network will at least intend to engage in those behaviors. Conversely, if the group is opposed to the

## 18    James Hawdon

behaviors, there is a heightened probability that the individual will not engage in the behavior.

Given that citizens' intentions should be highly correlated with their future behaviors, knowing these would be vital for public health officials as they plan to implement mitigation strategies. If officials can predict early on if people are unlikely to engage in the behaviors that can mitigate the threat, they can revise their plans and pursue alternative strategies that are likely to be followed more closely and therefore mitigate the threat more effectively. Moreover, officials may be able to address beliefs about factors that are perceived to be barriers to enacting the behavior or inform people about the relative risks and benefits of engaging in the behavior. Consequently, knowing peoples' plans can make policies more effective. As such, we focus on our respondents' plans to change their behaviors in this chapter. We will then see if these plans are related to their future behaviors in subsequent chapters. As noted, the individual's ability to control the behavior and the social norms about the behaviors influence the relationship between intentions and behaviors. Thus, we also analyze whether plans to change behaviors at the beginning of the pandemic are related to actual changed behaviors later in the pandemic. Doing so can inform us about the extent to which people thought they were able to control their behaviors and implement their plans and the changing social attitudes about those behaviors.

We now turn to the social context in which our respondents made their plans. As proposed by TPB, the information available to the respondents about the threat they faced should influence their intentions (Ajzen & Fishbein, 1980; Fishbein & Ajzen, 1975). Specifically, we focus on the toll the virus was extracting at the beginning of the pandemic in our two nations and how the relative threat influenced the extent to which people were concerned. We then look at what specific behaviors people planned to change and how these plans varied cross-nationally. We conclude by investigating the relationship between what people thought caused the pandemic and their planned behavioral changes.

## The Cross-national Context of COVID-19

As noted, responses varied cross-nationally based on the severity and early onset of cases (Capano et al., 2020; Lofredo, 2020). It is also clear that public attitudes toward and concerns about COVID-19 and the mitigation practices being recommended and implemented varied cross-nationally. The two nations we examine provide examples of differing COVID-19 experiences, at least early in the pandemic. The United States reported its first case on January 21, 2020, while Finland reported its first case more than a month later, on February 26. Not only was the onset of the disease later in Finland than in the United States, the United States also began experiencing far greater caseloads and deaths. By the end of March, the United States had become the hardest hit nation in the world, with over 81,000 confirmed cases and more than 1,000 deaths (Taylor, 2021).

According to John Hopkins University CSSE COVID-19 Data (Dong et al., 2023) by the end of March, the 7-day rolling average of newly confirmed cases

Planned Behavioral Changes 19

per million people was 3.5 times higher in the United States than it was in Finland, and confirmed deaths per million people were over twice as high in the United States than in Finland (Ritchie et al., 2022). As large as these gaps were at the beginning of the pandemic, they only grew wider over the initial stages of the pandemic. The figures present data from the early stages of the pandemic (from late January 2020 to late November 2020), and these data illustrate that COVID-19 was being experienced differently in the two nations. First, as shown in Fig. 2.1, the 7-day rolling average of daily new cases per million residents surpassed 100 in the United States early in the pandemic and skyrocketed to over 600 cases per million by October. In Finland, however, the 7-day rolling average of new cases per million residents during this time never surpassed 111 cases per million residents.

Similarly, while confirmed daily deaths were just under 8 per million Americans by mid-April 2020, it was just over 3 per million residents in Finland (see Fig. 2.2). What these data show is that the pandemic was bad in Finland, but it was worse in the United States.

Our data confirm that concern about the virus reflected the differences in disease severity in the two nations.[1] When respondents were asked how worried they were about the pandemic, similar percentages in the two nations expressed little concern (5.7% of Americans compared to 7.8% of Finns). Nearly three of four Finnish respondents said they were "slightly concerned," while only 38.9% of Americans expressed slight concern. Instead, Americans were far more likely to say they were "very concerned," with over half of American respondents reporting this level of concern. In comparison, approximately three times more Americans said they were very concerned than did Finnish respondents (see Fig. 2.3).

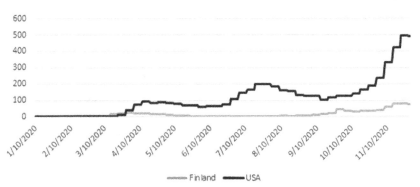

Fig. 2.1. New COVID-19 Cases Per Million Residents. *Source*: John Hopkins University CSSE COVID-19 data: https://github.com/CSSEGISandData/COVID-19.

---

[1]The analyses in this chapter are all limited to Wave I data since we are concerned with perceptions at the beginning of the pandemic.

20  James Hawdon

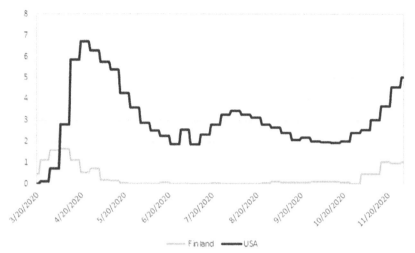

Fig. 2.2. New COVID-19 Deaths Per Million Residents. *Source*: John Hopkins University CSSE COVID-19 data: https://github.com/CSSEGISandData/COVID-19.

These differing levels of concern are striking. While the overwhelming number of citizens in both nations were concerned about the pandemic and the uncertain future it was causing, concern among Finns was disproportionately "slight" while concern among Americans was disproportionately higher. It is telling that at the time, fewer than one-in-five Finnish respondents said they were very concerned about the pandemic.

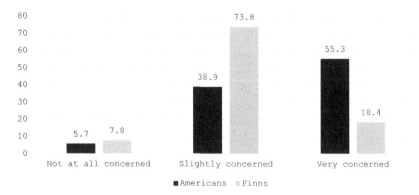

Fig. 2.3. Percent Residents Expressing Varying Levels of Concern About the Pandemic.

## Planned Behavioral Changes for Dealing with the Pandemic

The differences in levels of concern about the pandemic expressed by the citizens of each nation can help us understand other cross-national differences in attitudes toward and plans for dealing with the pandemic. Respondents were asked how likely they would engage in a variety of behaviors because of the pandemic, and several cross-national differences can be observed in their answers. We asked how likely they were to engage in 11 different behaviors because of the pandemic, and Fig. 2.4 reports the percentage of Americans and Finns who said they were likely or very likely to engage in each of the behaviors.[2]

As seen in Fig. 2.4, a few behaviors were reported by a majority of both Americans and Finns. For example, over 60% of respondents in both nations said that they were likely to avoid public gatherings in the future, and a majority of both Americans and Finns said they were likely to travel less often because of the pandemic. Not only did most respondents in both nations report plans to change these behaviors in the future, but the percentage also reporting such plans were

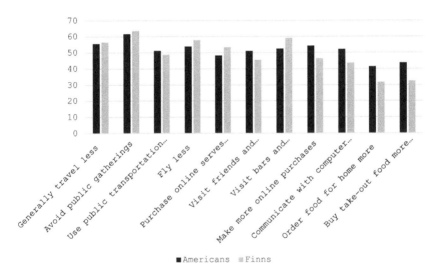

Fig. 2.4. Percent Residents Expressing Likelihood of Engaging in Various Behaviors.

---

[2]The differences between the two countries are not statistically significant for general travel, avoiding public gatherings, and using public transportation. The differences between the countries are statistically significant for the other behaviors at the $p < 0.05$ level (fly less often), $p < 0.01$ level (purchase online services and visit friends and relatives), and $p < 0.001$ level (visit bars, make online purchases, use computer, order food for home, and buy take-out).

## 22    James Hawdon

similar in both nations. The only other behaviors that were mentioned by a majority of both American and Finnish respondents were flying less and visiting bars and restaurants less; however, unlike plans for general travel and public gatherings, the cross-national differences in these behaviors were significantly different. For both flying less and visiting bars and restaurants less often, Finnish respondents were more likely than were American respondents to say they planned to adopt these behaviors. Compared to Americans, Finns were also more likely to say they would purchase online services such as movies, as over half of Finnish respondents (53.3%) reported they were likely to do this while slightly less than half of Americans (48.2%) said they were likely to purchase more online services.

For the remaining behaviors, American respondents were more likely than were Finnish respondents to say they foresaw a change in their behavior. While a majority of Americans said that they were likely to visit friends and relatives less, make more online purchases, and use computer programs like Zoom or FaceTime for interpersonal communication, only about 45% of Finnish respondents said they were likely to make these changes. Finally, it is interesting that while less than half of respondents in both nations said they would order food for their home more often or buy more take-out food, the cross-national differences were most pronounced for these behaviors. Americans were more likely than were Finns to say they planned to engage in these behaviors in the future, and the differences between the two sets of citizens were substantial. Nearly 10% more Americans than Finns said they were likely to order food for their home more often (41.3% vs 31.7%). Similarly, while 43.7% of Americans said they were likely to buy more take-out food in the future, only 32.5% of Finnish respondents said this. This is the largest cross-national difference found in any of these behaviors.

## Changing Interactions Versus Changing Consumer Behaviors

To help make sense of these cross-national differences, we grouped the behaviors using a Principal Components Factor Analysis.[3] This technique resulted in two unique dimensions that reflect distinct categories of planned changes. The first reflected *planned changes to interactions* with the questions about avoiding public gatherings, using public transportation less, traveling less, flying less, visit bars and restaurants less often, and visit friends and relatives less often. The second factor reflected *planned changes to consuming behaviors* with the questions

---

[3]Principal Components Analysis (PCA) is a variable-reduction technique that takes many variables, such as the 11 behaviors here, and reduces them into a smaller number of factors or "components" using a linear combination of the variables. It results in a few indices that reflect unique underlying concepts that the variables measure. The resulting indices differ because how each variable is weighted varies so that those variables that all reflect a similar dimension of a concept are weighted heavily on one component and weighted far less heavily on the other components. Thus, it results in a few new variables that reflect latent concepts that can then be used in other analyses.

*Planned Behavioral Changes*    23

concerning using computer programs like Zoom and FaceTime more, purchasing online services more, making online purchases more, order food for home more often, and ordering take-out food more often.[4] These two components reflect two strategies for managing the pandemic and mitigating the risks posed by the virus. The first strategy is to limit interactions with people outside one's immediate family. Most of these interactions are likely related to leisure activities (visiting friends and family, going to bars and restaurants, avoiding crowds, and traveling). In contrast, the second strategy is to reduce the amount of time one spends in stores, at work, or in other commercial establishments. Thus, the first strategy involves changes in how one plans to engage in primary relations with relatively close associates, while the second involves changes in how one plans to engage in secondary relations.

Grouping the behaviors allows us to investigate if Americans and Finns preferred different strategies. Comparing the means for these two variables between the two nations, Finnish respondents were significantly more likely to say they planned to change their *interactions* with close associates in leisure activities than were Americans, while Americans were significantly more likely to report they planned to change their *consuming behaviors* and secondary relations.[5] These relationships are surprising given the strong communal bonds among Finns for which they are famous. For example, Finnish respondents rank 6th of 29 European nations that participated in the European Social Survey[6] in terms of saying it is important to be loyal to friends and devote oneself to people close to them. Finnish respondents were significantly more likely to say this than Europeans were ($p < 0.001$). They were also more likely than other Europeans participating in the survey to say that it was important to "have a good time," "try new and different things in life," "seek fun things that give pleasures," and "seek adventures and have an exciting life."[7] All of these values point to the importance Finns place on friends, travel, leisure, and adventure, which are some of the activities our Finnish respondents said they were planning to limit in the future. Conversely, Americans being more likely than Finns to say they would alter their consuming behaviors as a strategy for avoiding the deadly COVID-19 virus is probably less surprising. Americans are known to be passionate about consumption, as the United States has the highest levels of per household disposable income and expenditure in the world (Euromonitor International, 2017), and saying they were more likely to engage in e-commerce does not imply they would purchase less

---

[4]The two-factor solution accounted for 64.37% of the variance in the 11 items. Communalities ranged from 0.513 to 0.733. Factor loadings from PCA are reported in the Appendix.

[5]Mean difference in change interactions ($T = 2.57$; $p = 0.010$). Mean difference in consuming behaviors ($T = 6.32$; $p < 0.001$).

[6]ESS Round 9: European Social Survey Round 9 Data (2018).

[7]$T$-tests were performed comparing Finns with all others in the sample. All differences were significant at the $p < 0.001$ except for the importance of seeking adventures and having an exciting life, which was significant at $p = 0.012$.

**24**   *James Hawdon*

goods or fewer services. Instead, it simply means they were planning to change *how* they consume.

Perhaps these differences reflect planned changes for the behaviors each nation's citizens engage in the most and therefore they feel put them most at risk for contracting the virus. That is, if Finnish citizens are typically more likely than Americans to visit friends, travel, and go to bars and restaurants, then they may be more willing to change these behaviors since they do them so frequently. Similarly, if Americans are most at risk of contracting the virus because they so frequently go shopping, eat in restaurants, and spend time in work meetings, they may be more willing than Finns are to curtail these behaviors and purchases goods and services online instead. While this is a possible explanation for these cross-national differences, we need to move beyond a bivariate analysis to investigate these differences further.

## Planned Changes and Beliefs About the Pandemic's Causes

One factor that could logically explain people's plans to change certain behaviors is their beliefs about what led to the pandemic. In the language of TPB, beliefs about what caused the pandemic would likely influence perceived behavioral controls as well as social norms. So, we asked people how much they thought a variety of possible causes of the pandemic contributed to it. Specifically, respondents were asked if they agreed or disagreed that immigration and migration, weak societal restrictions, leisure travel, and ineffective political decision-making contributed to the pandemic's outbreak and spread. Using these to predict if people planned to change their *interactions*, we find believing that these potential causes led to the pandemic significantly increased the likelihood of saying one would change their *interactions* to mitigate the pandemic's potential threat. Importantly, once these are entered into the model, there is no longer a statistically significant difference between the countries' residents.[8] Thus, differences in beliefs of what caused the pandemic between Americans and Finns mediate or erase the previously observed national differences in these plans. As will be discussed in Chapter 3, Finns were much more likely than Americans to believe that immigration, ease of leisure travel, and lack of social restrictions were contributing factors to the pandemic, and these factors were significant predictors of planning to change one's interactions.[9] Thus, national differences in the belief about the

---

[8]The model explains 4.5% of the variance in plans to change one's interactions to mitigate the effect of the pandemic. The slope coefficients for poor political decisions, lack of social restrictions, ease of leisure travel, and immigration were 0.127, 0.194, 0.235, and 0.080, respectively. The first three coefficients were significant at the $p \leq 0.001$ level, while believing immigration contributed to the pandemic was significant at the $p = 0.04$ level. Country was no longer statistically significant ($p = 0.606$).

[9]The differences in beliefs about contributing factors between the countries were significant for immigration, ease of leisure travel, and lack of social restrictions. Finns were more likely than Americans to believe immigration ($T = 4.99$; $p < 0.001$), ease of leisure travel ($T = 20.192$; $p < 0.001$), and the lack of social restrictions ($T = 7.95$;

*Planned Behavioral Changes* **25**

cause of the pandemic is what drove the national differences in plans for changing *interactions* as a strategy to manage the pandemic's threats.

While taking people's beliefs about what caused the pandemic into consideration explains the observed differences between Americans and Finns in terms of their plans to change their interactions because of the pandemic, this was not the case when trying to explain the national differences in plans to change *consuming behaviors* to mitigate the pandemic's threats. While those who believed the pandemic was caused by the lack of social restrictions were more likely to say they would change their consuming behaviors because of the pandemic, the national differences remain even after controlling this and the other factors.[10] Americans were still significantly more likely than were Finns to say they would rely on virtual means of consuming.

These cross-national differences in plans to change one's consuming behaviors hold even after we control demographic factors and how worried one was about the pandemic. Unsurprisingly, the more one was worried about the pandemic, the more likely they were to say they planned to change their consuming behaviors. Similarly, those with a college degree were more likely than those with less education to say they would change their consuming behaviors, but females and older respondents were less likely to say they would change their consuming behaviors than were males and younger respondents. Yet, these factors do not mediate the relationship between country and plans for future consumer behaviors. Compared to Finnish respondents, Americans were still significantly more likely to say they planned to purchase more online services and goods, order food for home more often, and order take-out food more often.

Again, a plausible explanation for these cross-national differences is the sheer volume of e-commerce in the United States. The United States is the leading e-commerce country with a well-established environment for such activities (Hwang et al., 2006). Indeed, in 2020, the United States was second to China in terms of e-commerce sales (eMarketer, 2022), and the United States ranks second to the United Kingdom in terms of e-commerce expenditures per capita (Ecommerce Foundation, 2020; Frisby, 2021). Perhaps this is why Americans were more likely to say they would engage in even more e-commerce as a way of

---

$p < 0.001$) contributed to the pandemic. While Americans were more likely than Finns to believe that ineffective politics contributed to the pandemic, the difference was not statistically significant ($T = -0.281$; $p = 0.779$). The effect sizes for ease of travel (Cohen's $D = 0.517$) and lack of social restrictions (Cohen's $D = 0.203$) were moderate, while the effect size for immigration was weak (Cohen's $D = 0.128$). The effective size for ineffective politics was very weak (Cohen's $D = 0.007$).

[10]Believing the lack of social restrictions led to the pandemic was significantly related to plans to change one's consuming behaviors ($b = 0.165$; $p < 0.001$); however, poor politic decision-making ($p = 0.241$), ease of leisure travel ($p = 0.504$), and immigration ($p = 0.075$) were not significant predictors of plans to change consuming behaviors. Country was also significant at the $p < 0.001$ level, with Americans being more likely than Finns to say they planned to change their behavior ($b_{USA} = 0.255$). The model accounted for 2.5% of the variance in plans to change consuming behaviors.

avoiding the threats posed by the pandemic. They already do these things a lot; doing them more would not require a tremendous amount of change. Moreover, as noted previously, the changes Americans said they were likely to make only altered *how* they were purchasing goods and services; these changes did not require Americans to change *how much* they purchased. As argued by the TPB, the intention to engage in a behavior is influenced by the value people place on the behavior, the ease with which it can be performed, and the norms concerning the behavior. This theory would therefore predict that Americans would say they intended to change their consuming behaviors because consumption is clearly valued, consuming remotely rather than in person is easy to do, and the norms of avoiding crowds during a pandemic were likely favorable at the time.

## Concluding Thoughts: How Much Change?

The initial stages of the pandemic undoubtedly led to shock and concern. As cases and deaths mounted, people assessed how to best protect themselves and their loved ones. The overwhelming majority of our respondents said they would likely change at least 1 of the 11 behaviors about which we asked them. Only 13.4% of respondents said they were unlikely to change any behavior; nearly as many (11.8%) said they were likely to change all 11 behaviors. Interestingly, these extremes also varied by nation, but Americans were more likely than Finns to say they were likely to change no behaviors as well as more likely than Finns to say they were likely to change all of the behaviors. Fig. 2.5 presents these data.

Perhaps this polarization in early plans for coping with the pandemic foreshadowed what we now know happened in terms of polarized responses to mask wearing, mandated lockdowns, and vaccinations. We will revisit these issues in later chapters.

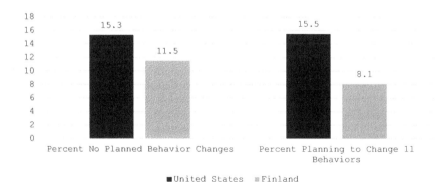

Fig. 2.5. Percent Residents Reporting Plans to Change None of the Listed Behaviors and Percent Planning to Change All 11 Listed Behaviors by Country.

## References

Ajzen, I. (1991). The theory of planned behavior. *Organizational Behavior and Human Decision Processes, 50*(2), 179–211.

Ajzen, I., & Fishbein, M. (1980). *Understanding attitudes and predicting social behavior.* Prentice Hall.

Albarracin, D., Johnson, B. T., Fishbein, M., & Muellerleile, P. A. (2001). Theories of reasoned action and planned behavior as models of condom use: A meta-analysis. *Psychological Bulletin, 127*(1), 142–161.

Capano, G., Howlett, M., Darryl, D. S. L., Ramesh, M., & Goyal, N. (2020). Mobilizing policy (in)capacity to fight COVID-19: Understanding variations in state responses. *Policy and Society, 39*(3), 285–308. https://doi.org/10.1080/14494035.2020.1787628

Dong, E., Du, H., & Gardner, L. (2023). An interactive web-based dashboard to track COVID-19 in real time. *The Lancet Infectious Diseases, 20*(5), 533–534. https://doi.org/10.1016/S1473-3099(20)30120-1

Dyer, P. (2021). *Policy and institutional responses to COVID-19: New Zealand.* Brookings Institute. https://www.brookings.edu/research/policy-and-institutional-responses-to-covid-19-new-zealand/#:~:text=From%20a%20global%20perspective%2C%20New,borders%20and%20its%20domestic%20economy

Ecommerce Foundation. (2020). *Global B2C ecommerce report.* www.ecommercefoundation.org/reports.

eMarketer. (2022). *Top 10 countries, ranked by retail ecommerce sales, 2020 & 2021.* https://www.emarketer.com/chart/242909/top-10-countries-ranked-by-retail-ecommerce-sales-2020-2021-billions-change

ESS Round 9: European Social Survey Round 9 Data. (2018). *Data file edition 3.1.* NSD – Norwegian Centre for Research Data, Norway – Data Archive and distributor of ESS data for ESS ERIC. https://doi.org/10.21338/NSD-ESS9-2018

Euromonitor International. (2017). *Ranked: Top 10 countries by consumer expenditure.* https://www.euromonitor.com/article/consumer-expenditure-top-10-countries

Finnish Government. (2020). *Information and advice on the coronavirus.* https://valtioneuvosto.fi/en/information-on-coronavirus

Fishbein, M., & Ajzen, I. (1975). *Belief, attitude, intention, and behavior: An introduction to theory and research.* Addison-Wesley.

Frisby, J. (2021). *The world's biggest online spenders revealed.* https://www.websitebuilderexpert.com/blog/worlds-biggest-online-spenders/

Giritli Nygren, K., & Olofsson, A. (2020). Managing the Covid-19 pandemic through individual responsibility: The consequences of a world risk society and enhanced ethopolitics. *Journal of Risk Research, 23*(7–8), 1031–1035.

Hale, T., Angrist, N., Hale, A. J., Kira, B., Majumdar, S., Petherick, A., Phillips, T., Sridhar, D., Thompson, R. N., Webster, S., & Zhang, Y. (2021). Government responses and COVID-19 deaths: Global evidence across multiple pandemic waves. *PLoS One, 16*(7), e0253116.

Hwang, W., Jung H. S., & Salvendy, G. (2006). Internationalisation of e-commerce: a comparison of online shopping preferences among Korean, Turkish and US populations. *Behaviour & Information Technology, 25*(1), 3–18. https://doi.org/10.1080/01449290512331335636

Lofredo, M. P. (2020). Social cohesion, trust, and government action against pandemics. *Eubios Journal of Asian and International Bioethics, 30*(4), 182–188.

Nguyen, M. N., Potvin, L., & Otis, J. (1997). Regular exercise in 30-to 60-year-old men: Combining the stages-of-change model and the theory of planned behavior to identify determinants for targeting heart health interventions. *Journal of Community Health, 22*(4), 233–246.

## 28 *James Hawdon*

Ritchie, H., Mathieu, E. Rodés-Guirao, L., Appel, C., Giattino, C., Ortiz-Ospina, E., Hasell, J., Macdonald, B., Dattani, S., & Roser, M. (2022). *Coronavirus pandemic (COVID-19)*. Our World in Data. https://ourworldindata.org/coronavirus#coronavirus-country-profile

Sedgwick, D., Hawdon, J., Räsänen, P., & Koivula, A. (2022). The role of collaboration in complying with COVID-19 health protective behaviors: A cross-national study. *Administration & Society, 54*(1), 29–56.

Taylor, D. B. (2021, March 17). A timeline of the coronavirus pandemic. *The New York Times*. https://www.nytimes.com/article/coronavirus-timeline.html

Welker K., Bennett, G. & Clark, D. (2020, April 2). *CDC recommends people wear cloth masks in public – But Trump says he won't*. https://www.nbcnews.com/news/us-news/u-s-expected-recommend-masks-americans-coronavirus-hotspots-n1175596

Chapter 3

# Which Factors Contributed to the COVID-19 Outbreak to Become a Global Pandemic?

*Pekka Räsänen and Aki Koivula*

*University of Turku, Finland*

### Abstract

The chapter is theoretically framed using theories of risk perception and work on the risk society. We aim at answering two fundamental questions: which factors did Americans and Finns considered to be the main reasons for the pandemic spread and were there differences in the perceptions of Americans and Finns at different points in the early stages of the pandemic. We compare the perceptions of several implicit causes ranging from the immigrants and migration to business travel, lack of citizen responsibility, and ineffective political decisions. Since social response to the COVID-19 pandemic were highly politicized in Western countries, and especially in the United States, our primary focus is on the effects of political party preference. The findings show that the effects were strongest when analyzing the belief that migration and immigration played a role in the pandemic's cause and spread. In the United States, supporters of Republican Party were more likely to perceive migrants and immigration as a cause for pandemic. In Finland, supporters of the coalition of parties in power at the time were less likely to do so. Temporal changes in the effects were also detected. Specifically, political preference was a weaker predictor of Americans' perception in fall than it had been in the spring. Our findings highlight how citizens do not believe all news coverage and claims about the disease, but instead political beliefs and life experiences have an important filtering effect on

---

Perceptions of a Pandemic: A Cross-Continental Comparison of Citizen Perceptions, Attitudes, and Behaviors During COVID-19, 29–47

Copyright © 2025 by Pekka Räsänen and Aki Koivula

Published under exclusive licence by Emerald Publishing Limited

doi:10.1108/978-1-83608-624-620241003

## 30 Pekka Räsänen and Aki Koivula

their interpretations. These interpretations appear to be phenomena that can be controlled at the national level.

*Keywords*: Risk society; risk perceptions; political preferences; social response to health crises; COVID-19

## Introduction

In 2020, many countries around the world faced an exceptionally wide-ranging crisis as the new coronavirus (SARS-CoV-2) started to spread. The pandemic has created severe consequences at societal level, ranging from worsened health outcomes to economic turmoil. In retrospect, one key issue relates to the original causes and stages of the emergence of the pandemic. While it may still be too early to offer definitive interpretations, the phases of the pandemic's expansion seem to attract continuous research interest (e.g., Su et al., 2022; Zhang et al., 2022).

Indeed, the rapid spread of the coronavirus into a pandemic in early 2020 raises many questions. Policymakers and concerned citizens alike have made various statements seeking the root causes of the pandemic and assessing the trajectory of the virus' spread. The search for explanations has been rare and experts from various fields have regularly given contradictory comments in the media. Similar reflections on the root causes have followed many tragedies in the past.

Acts of terrorism, mass shootings, and other human-caused disasters have been examined from this perspective. As the events are often impossible to understand and deal with from a rational point of view, it is tempting to accept certain interpretations that may offer simple explanations that are easy to understand. The aim is also to maintain a psychological sense of control after tragedies (e.g., Cinti, 2015; Hanuscin, 2013; Lindström et al., 2010). We believe biological events, including infection outbreaks and pandemics, can be understood from this perspective.

Our approach is not new. Sociological literature has long talked about a risk society, where people are more easily sensitized to external risk and threat factors (e.g., Beck, 1992; Giddens, 1991). A key argument is that the uncertainties of everyday life are perceived as personal and that protection against them is seen as of primary importance for one's identity. People must deal first-hand with various threats, choices, and opportunities that were previously solvable, for example, in a family community or through arrangements based on social security networks.

This new situation implies a lowered risk tolerance, even though external risk and threat factors are perceived as quasi-normal phenomena. Research shows that citizens in Western countries are increasingly sensitive to external disturbances (e.g., Callens & Meuleman, 2017; Leiserowitz, 2005; Räsänen et al., 2012). It is likely that the risks inherent in interest rates have become a central phenomenon shaping everyday experience. Similarly, with the corona pandemic, risky social experiences may have become even more common than before.

*Factors Contributed to the COVID-19 Outbreak* **31**

In the public debate, the causes of the COVID-19 pandemic have been associated such factors as China's population size and Chinese eating habits, the free movement of people and goods, as well as actions related to the various stages of the contagion phase. Medical studies have attempted to explain the emergence and evolution of aggressively spreading viruses and have suggested ways to prevent pandemics (e.g., Rothan & Byrareddy, 2020; Shereen et al., 2020). However, most contributions have focused on the underlying cultural and regulatory phenomena, which has made it difficult to see the bigger picture of the spread of coronavirus infections into a global pandemic.

We believe that the key point is that neither expert opinion nor the public debate has tended to focus on any single cause as being more relevant than others. In the absence of accurate, and neutral, information, rumors and opinions have tended to foster fears and panic among the population. In many cases, the initial assumptions made by the media about the course of events are later proven to be incorrect. For example, initial claims about the mechanisms of coronavirus transmission, modes of spread, and risk factors for severe disease have changed over time. When knowledge is uncertain, the spread of rumors has been typical of previous respiratory outbreaks, such as the SARS epidemic that hit Asia in 2003 (Cinti, 2015; Parashar & Anderson, 2004).

This chapter examines citizen perceptions of the reasons for the spread of the coronavirus pandemic. We aim to provide answers to the following two questions. First, which factors did Americans and Finns consider to be the main factors contributing to the spread of the pandemic in spring and autumn 2020? Second, were there differences in the perceptions of population groups at different points of time?

Since social response to the COVID-19 pandemic was highly politicized in Western countries, our primary focus is on the effects of political preference. As we focus on two separate time points from the first year of pandemic, we try to understand changes in a situation where little was known about the disease's nature.

# Interpretations on the Evolution of the COVID-19 Pandemic

In the absence of comprehensive explanations for the evolution of the corona situation into a pandemic, societal understanding of the situation is incomplete. However, it is possible to classify the offered interpretations according to the emphasis placed on the different aspects of the various explanations. In the public debate, several explanations have been given for the evolution of the corona epidemic into a pandemic.

First, the movement of people across borders, for example, in connection with tourism, migration, and emigration, has been highlighted. At the global level, one of the main ways of preventing the spread of the pandemic has been to restrict cross-border traffic. This line of explanation has been evident especially in studies examining national authorities and political decisions. In mobility research, it has been noted that pandemic and government responses impacted both voluntary

## 32   Pekka Räsänen and Aki Koivula

and involuntary mobility (Martin & Bergmann, 2021). Although global emergency resulted in a decrease of traveling and migration, on some occasions cross-border return migration and within-border movement increased. Similar framework has also been popular in research focusing on social media contents. For instance, Choli and Kuss (2021) reviewed blame attributes of Twitter data during the initial stages of the outbreak. One of the main findings was that the users blamed national governments and political leaders for keeping the national borders open. Results also documented the popularity of various conspiracy theories among the users on the virus' origin (Choli & Kuss, 2021).

Second, alongside restrictions on international movement, the citizen protection against a pandemic has been given a lot of attention. We can refer to such actions as restrictive measures. Typically, these interpretations have focused on the success and failure of a variety of national and local policy-making measures. In Finland, for example, there were various restrictions on the activities of private companies and public institutions. During the initial phase, the country had the Emergency Powers Act in force from March 17, 2020, to June 15, 2020 (Parliament of Finland, 2022). During that period, gatherings of more than 10 people were banned except, for example, hobby games or restaurant visits. Border crossing points were closed, and controls were also introduced at the European Union's internal borders. Trains and airlines were significantly reduced, especially to international traffic. People's movement within the country was also regulated. At the level of everyday life, derogations from the working hours and annual leave laws for health and police personnel were allowed, and retired police officers could also be assigned to work. In health care, it was no longer necessary to provide cursory care within the earlier schedule. Later, educational institutions moved to distance learning, public service facilities were closed, and many service sector companies were restricted (Tiirinki et al., 2024).

Similar, although lighter, restrictive measures took place in the United States. On March 13, a national emergency was declared by the President (White House, 2022). Following this, strict travel restrictions from Schengen Europe and various countries become immediately effective for non-American citizens. However, most regulations regarding, for instance, stay-at-home orders, remote work and studying, and loosening requirements for getting loans, took place at state level. California was the first state to issue mandatory regulations to stay at home and health care prioritizations. While many states later issued similar measures, it was already in the spring of 2020, when discussions on reopening the economy started to emerge (Suh & Alhaery, 2022). These plans were either postponed or reversed in most states as the number of positive cases continued to rise in the country. When compared to Finland, most visible country-wide measures dealt clearly with economic support for private households and business. Government and institution measure in response to pandemic were oriented toward health care support and for vaccine development. Despite this, however, COVID-19 emergency declaration was effective in the United States for nearly 3 years.

Third, in addition to evaluating the actions of policymakers and governmental institutions, individuals were concerned about their fellow citizens' adherence to public health advice and carelessness in their daily behaviors. For instance, we can think of such actions as washing hands or the requirements of using masks or keeping social distance in public gatherings. Consequently, adherence with new pandemic-related social norms quickly evolved into a moral issue (Prosser et al., 2020), and those who did not comply with new norms were perceived as contributing to the worsening of the pandemic conditions (Bor et al., 2023). Perhaps the most important concern connects to self-quarantining when infected (e.g., Mutz & Gerke, 2021; Sedgwick et al., 2022).

There were notable differences between the protective measures in the United States and Finland during the different phases of pandemic. In the United States, using face masks and other protective measures became a political divide that symbolized the chaos of the national response to the pandemic. Attitudes toward shutting schools and offices, as well as other policies for controlling the spread of the virus, were quite different between the Republican and Democratic camps. Similar political divide was not visible in Finland. In addition, we may note that the regulations varied significantly between the American states. Likewise, mandatory restrictions and official recommendations were more comprehensive in Finland when compared to the United States.

The fourth factor contributing to the spread of the pandemic is the impact of various ecological, demographic, or other phenomena that go beyond the actions of individual states. These factors include food production and distribution practices, population growth, and, in general, various global phenomena such as trade and raw material supply arrangements. The most widely discussed phenomenon in international literature has been wildlife street markets, which provide with an inherent part of food distribution in many Asian and Middle East countries. In these markets, it is common to sell wild and farmed wildlife alive and under conditions in which different species can easily come in touch with each other. Since the beginning of the pandemic, it has been argued the origins of the SARS-CoV-2 virus can be traced to certain wild animals, especially to bats or armadillos (Worobey et al., 2022). While laboratory leak assumptions have also been prominent in the media, many commentaries argue that it is the continuous interaction with animals that made the rapid outbreak possible (Rozado, 2021). Naturally, the debate on the virus' origin is still ongoing, but live animal distribution is one possible factor contributing to the pandemic's rapid outbreak.

Our final classification of causes is linked to information sharing and the forms of online communication. The development of information networks and the intensification of information transmission are behind these causes. A key factor in the transmission of information is the internet and the explosion in the use of digital technologies, which are increasingly enabling people to access information about events in various parts of the world. At the same time, verifying the origin and accuracy of information has become more challenging (Borgman, 2010). There are already several studies on such topics as "fake news" and "infodemics" in international literature (Rocha et al., 2021). Generally, these terms refer to an overabundance of correct and incorrect information in the daily media landscape, which makes it difficult for individuals to process what is really going on. Main argument relying on these studies is that during the pandemic a significant amount of information about coronavirus has been shared online and other

## 34    Pekka Räsänen and Aki Koivula

medium, some of which were accurate and some not. Inaccurate information has led to COVID-19 fake news experiences for many citizens, which has prevented individuals from following accurate measures in their daily life. Given this, fake news can be considered as one of the possible sources for the development of global pandemic.

Naturally, there are many alternative ways of classifying causes that led to the emergence situation and to the spread of the pandemic. We believe these five explanations combine many of the phenomena that have been the subject of social debate.

## Differences in the Public Perceptions

We need to acknowledge that people may have varying perceptions of the causes of the pandemic because they have encountered different debates about the origins of the pandemic. As is well known, different people connect with each other in different ways and are accordingly influenced, for example, by the news and various online discussions. Routines in everyday life also vary, from consumption and employment to leisure activities. In the light of research on social interaction and everyday practices, the main social contacts people create are based on their shared similarities. Similarity is often based on a wide range of characteristics: age, sex, differences by educational groups, or lifestyle choices. The assumption is that similarities unite people and dissimilarities separate them. This also goes with perceptions and attitudes.

At the general level, we can talk about the differentiation of life experiences. This phenomenon has been characterized in literature as social closure, narrowing of contact surfaces, or emergence of social "bubbles" (e.g., Flaxman et al., 2016; Keipi et al., 2017). It is likely that during the corona pandemic, the differentiation of experiences has become more pronounced. This is due to the constraints imposed on social life, which limit physical mobility and drive people into more restricted everyday routines.

While the levels of interaction came down, many were also interacting less with others who did not share similar socio-economic backgrounds. The findings from different countries point to the fact that population segments were differently affected by the safety measures and regulations (e.g., Chowell & Mizumoto, 2020; Sedgwick et al., 2022; Wilska et al., 2020). This is why variation associated with basic demographic factors, such as age and sex, needs to be acknowledged when examining perceptions of the causes that led to the pandemic.

We may also note that the use of the internet and digital services has increased during the pandemic. Stay-at-home mandates, closure of restaurants, and cultural affairs had notable impact on citizen's normal social activities. Many started teleworking, and online communication with colleagues, friends, and relatives increased while physical meetings declined. Video conferencing and phone calls have become the primary modes of social interaction, especially in the early phases of the pandemic. This kind of shift took place across all age groups, especially among the more education population in both the United States and Finland (e.g., Dahiya et al., 2021; Farooq et al., 2021; OSF, 2021). As social media and other digital communication tools became crucial sources of information during the pandemic, educational groups adopted different use patterns or online communication.

We aim to compare the popularity of alternative explanations for COVID-19 pandemic by acknowledging individual and cross-country variation in the responses. Added to the effects of conventional background variables such as age, sex, and education, we believe it is also important to address respondents' political preference, which is rooted in the reference groups and social embeddedness of daily activities (Koivula, 2019). One's political preference arises from social environment, and the associated party may modify the networks to which the citizen is attached (e.g., Campbell et al., 1960; Zuckerman, 2005).

According to traditional views, supporters of the given parties are likely to contact politically similar citizens, forming politically similar networks that indirectly determine supporters' attitudes and behaviors (Lazarsfeld & Merton, 1954). This is nowadays an important notion as class voting has been common but has diminished in Western societies, while the influence of post-materialist values on political orientation has increased (Knutsen, 2017). Following this, political affiliation can be considered as a direct result of personal interest, the adoption of different cultural values, and worldviews. In this respect, we may argue that citizens use political parties as their reference groups in forming opinions, and party preference can also function in the opposite direction in relation to their own experiences, regarding for instance coronavirus pandemic.

## Data, Variables, and Analytic Technique

The aim of the analysis is to find out to what extent perceptions of the pandemic causes can be grouped against the socio-demographic background of respondents and to what extent there has been a temporal change in this distribution. Interpretations are made from a temporal reference setting. The central problem of previous research on the topic has concerned the use of cross-sectional data in perceiving and analyzing process-like phenomena. As is well known, in the light of data on a single point in time, it is not possible to assess the changes that have occurred in social reality.

We assume that there are differences between different population groups in how Americans and Finns view the spread of the coronavirus pandemic. Our analysis focuses on comparing differences between population groups by political preference. We consider party preferences as lens through which citizens evaluate the adequacy of COVID-19 explanations in relation to their own experiences and interpretations. In the American sample, the party preference variable is dichotomized between "Republican Party supporter" and "Other" as the United States Government was Republican at the time of data collection. In Finland, which is a multi-party country, the situation at the time of research was that the Government consisted of five parties: Social Democratic Party, Centre Party, Green League, Left Alliance, and Swedish People's Party. Preferences for these parties were labeled as "Government party supporter," and the remaining ones as "Other."

## 36 *Pekka Räsänen and Aki Koivula*

In addition, age, gender, and educational level are used as control variables. The background variables selected for analysis are those that can be thought to reflect differences in people's lifestyles in general. The underlying assumption is that respondents' assessments reflect the public debate on the causes of the emergence and spread of the pandemic. We also assume that there have been some changes in the views of Americans and Finns between spring and autumn 2020.

We examine changes according to the factors that are perceived to be the causes of the pandemic and the ways in which these perceptions vary both by population group and by time. Citizens' views on the causes of the pandemic are interpreted from two different perspectives. First, the different factors are examined in terms of their importance for the population in spring and autumn 2020. After this, based on this cross-sectional analysis, the differences in perceptions by political preference are compared using the merged data for spring and autumn. The dependent variables for the analysis include perceived causes of the pandemic. Specifically, we focus on if respondents believed migrants and immigration, weak social restrictions, a lack of civic responsibility, and wildlife street markets contributed to the coronavirus outback becoming a pandemic (see the Appendix for details). The primary independent variable is political preference. Specifically, this focused on being a member of the political party that was in power at the time (i.e., Republicans in the United States and the Government party in Finland). Control variables included sex, age, and education. The reader should consult the Appendix for details.

## Descriptive Analysis

In late 2019, the first cases of coronavirus found in China were reported worldwide. The popular public interpretation has been that the virus has been transmitted to humans from wild animals, but the laboratory origin of the virus had also been suspected. Initially, cases were concentrated in China and Asia, but as spring 2020 progressed, infections began to be found on all continents. By the autumn of 2020, Asia had all but escaped the pandemic, as the number of cases increased in Europe and especially in the United States.

The incidence of infections has been subject to large temporal variations. However, the detection of infection waves confounds with seasonal variation due to climatic variation and testing rates in the population. In Europe, for example, there was already talk of a second wave of the pandemic in autumn 2020, while the United States was still in the first wave. A key factor in the evolution of the pandemic situation has been that the surge in infection peaks was most pronounced in countries outside Asia. Since then, there have been many public interpretations of how, in China at least, actual infection rates have been grossly distorted downwards. Such speculation has been made about both the first and subsequent waves (e.g., Chowell & Mizumoto, 2020; Lau et al., 2020).

In this study, the population's views on the origin of the coronal pandemic are examined from the perspective of the first wave of infection in spring and the

## Factors Contributed to the COVID-19 Outbreak 37

second wave in autumn. As the data we use were collected in April and November 2020, the interpretations can be first mirrored in a general way with respect to the infection situations in our country at those times. This analysis is not so much about how individual respondents' views have changed over time but about the prevailing perception of the most and least important causes.

Fig. 3.1 shows the perceptions of the Finnish and American respondents in spring and autumn for each of the statements asked in the questionnaire. The observations from both rounds of the survey ($N$=6,073) are included. In the graphs, the experience of the causes of the pandemic is presented as a percentage of respondents who agree or strongly agree with the statement presented. It should be considered that the questionnaire's wording and statements may contain minor validity problems. It is not self-evident that all respondents have the same perception of the phenomena presented in the questionnaire. However, the statements concerning the different phenomena have been formulated as unambiguously as possible.

The graph shows that in autumn and spring, lack of citizen responsibility and wildlife street markets were the most frequently perceived cause of the pandemic. In spring, 69% of Finns agreed or strongly agreed that lack of civic responsibility contributed to the spread of the coronavirus into a pandemic. In autumn, 72% agreed. In the United States, the shares were 56% for spring and 64% for autumn.

In the case of wildlife street markets, it is interesting to note that the proportions are significantly lower for the United States. In the spring, 48% felt that

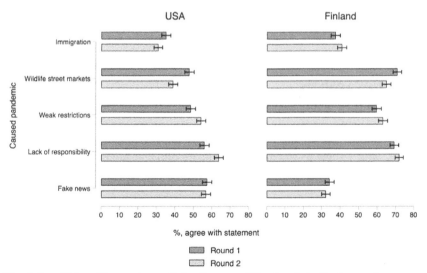

Fig. 3.1. Citizen Perceptions of the Causes of Pandemic in Spring and Autumn 2020, Shares of Agreement (%) and Margins of Error (95% Confidence Level).

*38   Pekka Räsänen and Aki Koivula*

wildlife street markets had a significant impact, and this proportion was a further nine percentage points lower in the autumn (39%). In Finland, on the other hand, 71% viewed wildlife street markets as worthy cause for the pandemic. By fall, the share dropped by six percentage points to 65%.

In the United States, the proportions were 35% in spring and 31% in autumn. Among the factors related to political decisions, perceptions were also different between the countries. Weak social restrictions were perceived as a significant factor by 60% of Finns in spring and 63% in autumn. In the United States, the shares were lower with 49% for spring and 54% for autumn.

It is also noteworthy that broad factors related to social conditions or global problems were perceived as having a relatively minimal impact on the pandemic. In Finland, 38% perceived migrants and immigrants in spring and 41% in the autumn as influencing factors for the pandemic. In addition, false information spread on the internet, or "fake news," showed clearly different findings for the countries. In Finland, 34% viewed that such information played a role in spring, and 32% in autumn. In the American data, the shares were significantly higher with 58% for spring and 57% for autumn.

If we compare the situation in spring and autumn for all respondents, with an exception for wildlife street markets, experiences seem to have changed little. Indeed, the confidence intervals (95% CI) shown in Fig. 3.1 indicate that the differences between spring and autumn remain small. However, we can witness smaller changes for weak social restrictions in the United States and migrants and immigration for both countries.

Next, we turn to examine how these five items are associated with respondents' political preferences. We look at what kind of differences there were between the countries and examine the differences in responses in the spring and fall of 2020. In addition, we test the possible effects of respondents' age, sex, and level of education.

## Predictive Analysis

In the predictive analysis, we used regression models to assess the effects of independent variables on perceptions of causes that contributed to the COVID-19 outbreak becoming a pandemic. Analyses are reported as linear probability coefficients, which allow us to efficiently compare different models with each other (for details, see Breen et al., 2018). The models in the tables compare probabilities among different population groups for the United States and Finland. The parameter estimates report average differences in the probabilities in percentages between value 1 ("agrees") and 0 ("disagrees") against the reference category. In addition, standard deviations are given in parentheses.

First, we included the main effects of political preference, each control variable and time of data collection (second round). Table 3.1 gives findings for the American sample, in which "Other than Republican" is treated as reference category. We can see that those supporting the Republicans are 15% more likely than others to perceive migrants and immigration as cause for pandemic.

*Factors Contributed to the COVID-19 Outbreak*  **39**

Table 3.1.  Predicted Perceptions of the Causes of Pandemic in the United States.

| Variables | Migrants and Immigration | Wildlife Street Markets | Weak Restrictions | Lack of Responsibility | Fake News |
|---|---|---|---|---|---|
| Republican Party supporter | 0.148*** (0.018) | 0.015 (0.019) | –0.062** (0.019) | –0.028 (0.019) | –0.068** (0.019) |
| Age | –0.002*** (0.001) | –0.001 (0.001) | –0.000 (0.001) | 0.001* (0.001) | 0.001* (0.001) |
| Female | –0.077*** (0.017) | –0.054** (0.018) | –0.029 (0.018) | –0.027 (0.018) | –0.014 (0.018) |
| College degree | –0.031 (0.017) | 0.102*** (0.018) | 0.063*** (0.018) | 0.066*** (0.018) | 0.074*** (0.018) |
| Second round (fall) | –0.044** (0.017) | –0.082*** (0.018) | 0.059** (0.018) | 0.082*** (0.018) | –0.002 (0.018) |
| Observations | 3,035 | 3,035 | 3,035 | 3,035 | 3,035 |

\*\*\* $p<0.001$, \*\* $p<0.01$, \* $p<0.05$.
*Note*: Probabilities of agreement with Standard errors in parentheses.

The probabilities are also six to seven percentage points lower for Republican supporters when weak social restrictions and online fake news are examined. There are no statistical differences in wildlife street markets or lack of citizen responsibility.

As for control variables, education is a significant predictor for all items except migrants and immigration. Those with at least a college degree are more likely than others to view wildlife street markets, weak restrictions, lack of responsibility, and fake news as factors contributing to pandemic. The table also shows that age and sex are significant predictors. In fact, each year of respondent's age is associated with a 0.2% drop of probability in perceiving migrants as a cause contributing to the pandemic. The probability for females compared to males is almost 8% lower in case of migrants and immigration, and over 5% in wildlife street markets.

Here, we can also notice that perceptions changed significantly between spring and fall in the United States. Weak restrictions and lack of responsibility were more likely seen as causes contributing to pandemic in fall. On the contrary, migrants and immigration, and wildlife street markets, were more likely causes in spring, when the expansion of the pandemic was just in its initial phase.

Table 3.2 shows regression models for Finnish sample. "Opposition party supporter" is treated as reference category in the examination of political preference. The first notion is that political preference is clearly significant for migrants and

**40** *Pekka Räsänen and Aki Koivula*

immigration and internet fake news. Those who support government parties are 15% less likely than opposition supporters to consider migrants and immigration as a contributing cause to pandemic. In the case of fake news, the effect is opposite with seven percentage points increased difference. Political preference is a weak predictor of other items. We consider these findings to be in line with American data. This is because the Finnish Government consisted predominately of left-wing parties (in contrast to right-wing Republican regime of the United States).

Sex is a significant predictor of wildlife street markets, weak restrictions, and lack of citizen responsibility. Females were more likely to perceive these items as significant factors contributing to the pandemic, ranging from five to eight percentage point differences compared to males. Age is significant for the lack of responsibility and fake news. Years of age increase the probability of viewing the lack of responsibility a significant factor, whereas we can witness a decline in the case of fake news. There are also educational differences between the two items. Those with college degrees are 10% less likely than others to consider migrants and immigration as a contributing factor to pandemic. On the other hand, college degree increases likelihood to perceive wildlife street market as a contributing factor with almost 5%.

Some of the perceptions changed significantly between spring and fall. However, there were not as many changes as in the United States. Also in Finland, wildlife street markets were more likely to be considered a cause of the pandemic

Table 3.2. Predicted Perceptions of the Causes of Pandemic in Finland.

| Variables | Migrants and Immigration | Wildlife Street Markets | Weak Restrictions | Lack of Responsibility | Fake News |
|---|---|---|---|---|---|
| Government party supporter | –0.152*** (0.018) | 0.035* (0.018) | –0.038* (0.018) | 0.013 (0.017) | 0.066** |
| Age | 0.001 (0.001) | 0.001** (0.001) | 0.000 (0.001) | 0.002*** (0.001) | –0.003*** (0.001) |
| Female | –0.016 (0.017) | 0.059*** (0.017) | 0.046** (0.018) | 0.079*** (0.016) | 0.015 (0.017) |
| College degree | –0.104*** (0.018) | 0.045** (0.017) | –0.021 (0.018) | 0.009 (0.017) | 0.002 (0.017) |
| Second round (fall) | 0.035* (0.017) | –0.058*** (0.017) | 0.034 (0.018) | 0.028 (0.016) | –0.022 (0.017) |
| Observations | 3,073 | 3,073 | 3,073 | 3,073 | 3,073 |

*** $p<0.001$, ** $p<0.01$, * $p<0.05$.
*Note*: Probabilities of agreement with standard errors in parentheses.

Factors Contributed to the COVID-19 Outbreak    41

in the spring of 2020. Added to this, the likelihood of seeing migrants and immigration as a notable factor increased slightly in fall (although the effect remains statistically almost significant).

Finally, we looked more closely at the effect of political preference in spring and fall. In other words, we examined whether there really was a change in the effects between the two measurement points in the United States and Finland. To accomplish this, we added the two-way interaction term between time point and party affiliation to the previous models. This enabled us also to consider the impact of age, sex, and educational level of the respondents. Fig. 3.2 illustrates the predicted probabilities between 0.0 and 0.8 for supporters of Republican/government parties at both measurement points after adjusting for control variables.

In the American data, results indicated that the effect of political preference for migrants and immigration, weak restrictions, and fake news failed to hold from spring to fall. Those supporting Republicans saw these factors of less importance in fall. The drop was statistically significant (at the level of $p<0.01$) for each of these items. The probabilities also weakened for other causes, but these changes failed to be statistically significant. The Finnish data did not show significant changes in the effect of political preference. Weak restrictions showed the only change that came close to statistical significance. Government supporters were slightly more likely to perceive weak restrictions as a contributing factor to pandemic in fall. The Appendix Table AI shows the full models for both countries with the added interaction term.

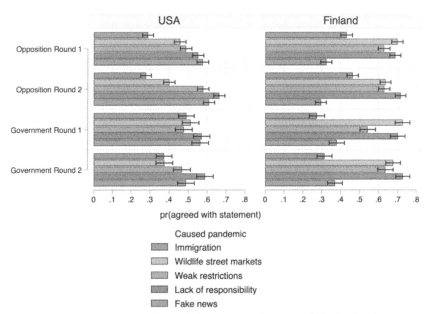

Fig. 3.2.   Predicted Perceptions of the Causes of Pandemic in Spring (Round 1) and Autumn (Round 2) by Political Preference. Probabilities of Agreement with Margins of Errors.

## 42 *Pekka Räsänen and Aki Koivula*

## Discussion

Attempts to offer definite explanations in ambiguous situations come with huge dangers. This is evident when addressing notable social risks such as the recent COVID-19 pandemic. Despite this, we have witnessed several interpretations on the origin of the coronavirus and the development of the pandemic. This chapter examined the experiences of Americans and Finns regarding different societal factors influencing the spread of the pandemic. Five alternative statements were compared in the spring and autumn of 2020. With few exceptions, the population responses were similar in both points of time.

The responses indicate that the most common perceptions of the causes are related to the lack of citizen responsibility and weak restrictive measures. In contrast, misinformation spread through information networks, or fake news, or migration and immigration were not perceived as common causes. The only notable difference between the countries was related to the role of wildlife street markets. In the beginning of the pandemic, regulating wildlife gateways was seen as one of the key measures for managing the situation (e.g., Roe et al., 2020; Watsa, 2020). Our results showed that wildlife street markets were considered as a common factor in Finland but not in the United States. In general, however, the causes that led to the pandemic were not perceived as a global phenomenon that cannot be easily influenced but rather as a phenomenon that can be controlled by national solutions. The responses highlight the importance of civic responsibility.

The analysis of differences in perceptions between different population groups was carried out by examining the statements according to political preference. Age, sex, and level of education served as control variables, which also influence the interpretations of the causes. The effect of political preferences was notable in both countries (see Tables 3.1 and 3.2). Perhaps as expected, the effects were strongest when explaining perceptions on migration and immigration. In the United States, supporters of the Republican Party were more likely to perceive migrants and immigration as a cause for pandemic. In Finland, supporters of Government parties were less likely to do so. Temporal changes in the effects were also detected, some of which were notably significant in the United States. Political preference was a weaker predictor of Americans' perception in the fall.

Our findings underline previous studies suggesting that citizens do not adopt all news coverage and claims about the disease as such (Qazi et al., 2020). Rather, political beliefs and various life experiences have an important filtering effect for interpretations. It is also necessary to acknowledge that views on the causes of pandemic can change over time, sometimes even in a very short period. The coronavirus pandemic has generated widespread debate on various media platforms and information on the disease has been highly fragmented. In this sense, our findings continue to have significance. Incorrect and misleading information about the causes of the pandemic continues to circulate in broadcast and social media (Orso et al., 2020). As for today, there is no consensus on the origins or trajectory of the pandemic, and the views of citizens in the United States and Finland cannot be interpreted in terms of a single culture. The uneven spread of coronavirus between countries also means that people have different experiences of the disease. People's views on the necessary and correct measures to contain the pandemic will change over time. For example, the means that dominate public debate and social media may gain widespread support in public perceptions. In this context, it is worth recalling that there is mixed research evidence on the actual effectiveness of various containment measures (e.g., Su et al., 2022; Suh & Alhaery, 2022). It follows that risk perceptions are partly different among population groups and may change over time.

Naturally, several problems must be considered when interpreting the results presented in this chapter. Most notably, the mechanisms of the causes that led to the pandemic were not defined in more detail. As a result, respondents may have perceived them in different ways, which may have influenced the results. One respondent may have argued that the phenomenon was the root cause of the spread of the virus. Another may have looked at the issue primarily as an extension of the epidemic level to the pandemic level. These types of problems always remain partially unresolved in survey research. Despite this, however, they should not be seen as an obstacle to the use of the results but only as factors limiting the interpretations made based on our findings.

## Conclusion

Preceding research clearly shows that many daily activities such as consumption practices and social interaction declined both in Finland and in the United States during the pandemic (e.g., Sedgwick et al., 2022; Wilska et al., 2020). In addition, expert views on the causes of pandemic have varied, along with various broadcast news reports and social media discussions. This is why the citizen interpretations about the underlying causes are often contradictory as they partly reflect those issues imposed by public authorities, official recommendations, and individuals. Explanations of the pandemic become more diverse as arguments spread among different population groups.

It is likely that the views of Finns and Americans will continue to vary over time and among population groups in the future. However, with reliable research data and effective research communication, the flow of verified information can be improved. There is currently a lack of cross-nationally comparative research data on citizens' interpretations and attitudes toward pandemics.

It is impossible to assess to what extent the interpretations based on the data collected in spring and autumn 2020 are still reliable. The deaths, exposures, and potential exposures associated with coronavirus infections have been the subject of intense media, expert, and everyday discourse for more than a year. This can only lead to the conclusion that more research on the aftermath of COVID-19 pandemic is required.

## 44 Pekka Räsänen and Aki Koivula

# References

Beck, U. (1992). From industrial society to the risk society: Questions of survival, social structure and ecological enlightenment. *Theory, Culture & Society*, 9(1), 97–123.

Bor, A., Jørgensen, F., Lindholt, M. F., & Petersen, M. B. (2023). Moralizing the COVID-19 pandemic: Self-interest predicts moral condemnation of other's compliance, distancing, and vaccination. *Political Psychology*, 44(2), 257–279.

Borgman, C. L. (2010). *Scholarship in the digital age: Information, infrastructure, and the internet.* MIT Press.

Breen, R., Karlson, K. B., & Holm, A. (2018). Interpreting and understanding logits, probits, and other nonlinear probability models. *Annual Review of Sociology*, 44, 39–54.

Callens, M. S., & Meuleman, B. (2017). Do integration policies relate to economic and cultural threat perceptions? A comparative study in Europe. *International Journal of Comparative Sociology*, 58(5), 367–391.

Campbell, A., Converse, P. E., Miller, W. E., & Stokes, D. E. (1960). *The American voter.* University of Chicago Press.

Choli, M., & Kuss, D. J. (2021). Perceptions of blame on social media during the coronavirus pandemic. *Computers in Human Behavior*, 124, 106895.

Chowell, G., & Mizumoto, K. (2020). The COVID-19 pandemic in the USA: What might we expect?. *The Lancet*, 395(10230), 1093–1094.

Cinti, S. (2015). Critical incident analysis, biological events, and the case of the 2009 H1N1 Influenza A pandemic. In R. W. Schwester (Ed.), *Handbook of critical incident analysis* (pp. 49–69). Routledge.

Dahiya, S., Rokanas, L. N., Singh, S., Yang, M., & Peha, J. M. (2021). Lessons from internet use and performance during COVID-19. *Journal of Information Policy*, 11, 202–221.

Farooq, A., Laato, S., Islam, A. N., & Isoaho, J. (2021). Understanding the impact of information sources on COVID-19 related preventive measures in Finland. *Technology in Society*, 65, 101573.

Flaxman, S., Goel, S., & Rao, J. M. (2016). Filter bubbles, echo chambers, and online news consumption. *Public Opinion Quarterly*, 80(S1), 298–320.

Giddens, A. (1991). *Modernity and self-identity: Self and society in the late modern age.* Stanford University Press.

Hanuscin, D. L. (2013). Critical incidents in the development of pedagogical content knowledge for teaching the nature of science: A prospective elementary teacher's journey. *Journal of Science Teacher Education*, 24(6), 933–956.

Jakonen, O., Luonila, M., Renko, V., & Kanerva, A. (2020). Katsaus koronan vaikutuksista taiteen ja kulttuurin alojen toimintaedellytyksiin ja kulttuuripolitiikkaan Suomessa. *Kulttuuripolitiikan Tutkimuksen Vuosikirja*, 5(1), 50–59.

Keipi, T., Näsi, M., Oksanen, A., & Räsänen, P. (2017). *Online hate and harmful content: Cross-national perspectives.* Routledge.

Knutsen, O. (2017). *Social structure, value orientations and party choice in western Europe.* Springer.

Koivula, A. (2019). *The choice is yours but it is politically tinged: The social correlates of political party preferences in Finland.* University of Turku.

Lau, H., Khosrawipour, V., Kocbach, P., Mikolajczyk, A., Ichii, H., Schubert, J., Bania, J., & Khosrawipour, T. (2020). Internationally lost COVID-19 cases. *Journal of Microbiology, Immunology and Infection*, 53(3), 454–458.

Lazarsfeld, P., & Merton, R. (1954). Friendship as social process: A substantive and methodological analysis. In M. Berger, T. Abel, & C. Page (Eds.), *Freedom and control in modern society* (pp. 18–66). Van Nostrand.

# Factors Contributed to the COVID-19 Outbreak 45

Leiserowitz, A. A. (2005). American risk perceptions: Is climate change dangerous? *Risk Analysis: An International Journal, 25*(6), 1433–1442.

Lindström, K., Nurmi, J., Oksanen, A., & Räsänen, P. (2010). Jokelan ja Kauhajoen asukkaiden arviot koulusurmien yhteiskunnallisista syistä. *Sosiologia, 47*, 4.

Martin, S., & Bergmann, J. (2021). (Im) mobility in the age of COVID-19. *International Migration Review, 55*(3), 660–687.

Mutz, M., & Gerke, M. (2021). Sport and exercise in times of self-quarantine: How Germans changed their behaviour at the beginning of the COVID-19 pandemic. *International Review for the Sociology of Sport, 56*(3), 305–316.

Official Statistics Finland (OSF). (2021). *Väestön tieto-ja viestintätekniikan käyttö* [verkkojulkaisu]. SSN=2341-8699. 2020. Tilastokeskus [viitattu: 14.4.2021].

Orso, D., Federici, N., Copetti, R., Vetrugno, L., & Bove, T. (2020). Infodemic and the spread of fake news in the COVID-19-era. *European Journal of Emergency Medicine, 27*(5), 327–328.

Parashar, U. D., & Anderson, L. J. (2004). Severe acute respiratory syndrome: Review and lessons of the 2003 outbreak. *International Journal of Epidemiology, 33*(4), 628–634.

Parliament of Finland. (2022). *Adoption of the Emergency Powers Act during the COVID-19 pandemic* [Online document]. Retrieved March 3, 2023, from https://www.eduskunta.fi/EN/naineduskuntatoimii/kirjasto/aineistot/kotimainen_oikeus/LATI/Pages/valmiuslain-kayttoonottaminen-koronavirustilanteessa.aspx

Prosser, A. M., Judge, M., Bolderdijk, J. W., Blackwood, L., & Kurz, T. (2020). 'Distancers' and 'non-distancers'? The potential social psychological impact of moralizing COVID-19 mitigating practices on sustained behaviour change. *British Journal of Social Psychology, 59*(3), 653–662.

Qazi, A., Qazi, J., Naseer, K., Zeeshan, M., Hardaker, G., Maitama, J. Z., & Haruna, K. (2020). Analyzing situational awareness through public opinion to predict adoption of social distancing amid pandemic COVID-19. *Journal of Medical Virology, 92*(7), 849–855.

Räsänen, P., Näsi, M., & Sarpila, O. (2012). Old and new sources of risk: A study of societal risk perception in Finland. *Journal of Risk Research, 15*(7), 755–769.

Rocha, Y. M., de Moura, G. A., Desidério, G. A., de Oliveira, C. H., Lourenço, F. D., & de Figueiredo Nicolete, L. D. (2021). The impact of fake news on social media and its influence on health during the COVID-19 pandemic: A systematic review. *Journal of Public Health, 31*, 1–10.

Roe, D., Dickman, A., Kock, R., Milner-Gulland, E. J., & Rihoy, E. (2020). Beyond banning wildlife trade: COVID-19, conservation and development. *World Development, 136*, 105121.

Rothan, H. A., & Byrareddy, S. N. (2020). The epidemiology and pathogenesis of coronavirus disease (COVID-19) outbreak. *Journal of Autoimmunity, 109*, 102433.

Rozado, D. (2021). Prevalence in news media of two competing hypotheses about COVID-19 origins. *Social Sciences, 10*(9), 320.

Sedgwick, D., Hawdon, J., Räsänen, P., & Koivula, A. (2022). The role of collaboration in complying with COVID-19 health protective behaviors: A cross-national study. *Administration & Society, 54*(1), 29–56.

Shereen, M. A., Khan, S., Kazmi, A., Bashir, N., & Siddique, R. (2020). COVID-19 infection: Origin, transmission, and characteristics of human coronaviruses. *Journal of Advanced Research, 24*, 91–98.

Su, R., Obrenovic, B., Du, J., Godinic, D., & Khudaykulov, A. (2022). COVID-19 pandemic implications for corporate sustainability and society: A literature review. *International Journal of Environmental Research and Public Health, 19*(3), 1592.

Suh, E., & Alhaery, M. (2022). Measuring reopening readiness: A universal COVID-19 index for U.S. states. *Library Hi Tech, 40*(2), 535–547.

## 46    Pekka Räsänen and Aki Koivula

Tiirinki, H., Sovala, M., Jormanainen, V., Goebeler, S., Parhiala, K., Tynkkynen, L. K., & Keskimäki, I. (2024). COVID-19 endemic phase in Finland: An analysis of health policies and vaccination strategy. *Health Policy and Technology*, *13*(1), 100800.

Watsa, M. (2020). Rigorous wildlife disease surveillance. *Science*, *369*(6500), 145–147.

Wilska, T. A., Nyrhinen, J., Tuominen, J., Šilinskas, G., & Rantala, E. (2020). Kulutus koronan aikana ja sen jälkeen: tutkimus COVID-19-epidemian rajoitustoimien vaikutuksesta kuluttajien käyttäytymiseen, taloudelliseen toimintaan ja hyvinvointiin. *Jyväskylän yliopiston kauppakorkeakoulun julkaisuja 2012/2020*. Jyväskylän yliopisto.

Worobey, M., Levy, J. I., Malpica Serrano, L., Crits-Christoph, A., Pekar, J. E., Goldstein, S. A., Rasmussen, A. L., Kraemer, M. U. G., Newman, C., Koopmans, M. P. G., Suchard, M. A., Wertheim, J. O., Lemey, P., Robertson, D. L., Garry, R. F., Holmes, R. F., Rambaut, A., & Andersen, K. G. (2022). The Huanan seafood wholesale market in Wuhan was the early epicenter of the COVID-19 pandemic. *Science*, *377*(6609), 951–959.

Zhang, Q., Gao, J., Wu, J. T., Cao, Z., & Dajun Zeng, D. (2022). Data science approaches to confronting the COVID-19 pandemic: A narrative review. *Philosophical Transactions of the Royal Society A*, *380*(2214), 20210127.

Zuckerman, A. S. (2005). *The social logic of politics: Personal networks as contexts for political behavior*. Temple University Press.

**Table AI.** Predicted Perceptions of the Causes of Pandemic in the United States and Finland.

| VARIABLES | The United States | | | | | Finland | | | | |
|---|---|---|---|---|---|---|---|---|---|---|
| | Migrants and Immigration | Wildlife Street Markets | Weak Restrictions | Lack of Responsibility | Fake News | Migrants and Immigration | Wildlife Street Markets | Weak Restrictions | Lack of Responsibility | Fake News |
| Republican/ government party supporter | 0.202*** (0.026) | 0.055* (0.027) | −0.011 (0.028) | 0.019 (0.027) | −0.013 (0.027) | −0.156*** (0.026) | 0.028 (0.025) | −0.085** (0.026) | 0.014 (0.024) | 0.056* (0.025) |
| 2. Round | −0.010 (0.020) | −0.057** (0.022) | 0.091*** (0.022) | 0.112*** (0.021) | 0.033 (0.022) | 0.032 (0.022) | −0.062** (0.021) | 0.001 (0.022) | 0.029 (0.020) | −0.028 (0.021) |
| Support party x 2.Round | −0.106** (0.036) | −0.081* (0.038) | −0.100** (0.039) | −0.094* (0.038) | −0.108** (0.038) | 0.009 (0.036) | 0.012 (0.035) | 0.093* (0.037) | −0.002 (0.034) | 0.019 (0.035) |
| Age | −0.002*** (0.001) | −0.001 (0.001) | −0.001 (0.001) | 0.001* (0.001) | 0.001* (0.001) | 0.001 (0.001) | 0.001** (0.001) | 0.000 (0.001) | 0.002*** (0.001) | −0.003** (0.001) |
| Female | −0.076*** (0.017) | −0.053** (0.018) | −0.027 (0.018) | −0.026 (0.018) | −0.012 (0.018) | −0.016 (0.017) | 0.059*** (0.017) | 0.045* (0.018) | 0.079*** (0.016) | 0.015 (0.017) |
| College degree | −0.032 (0.017) | 0.101*** (0.018) | 0.063*** (0.018) | 0.065*** (0.018) | 0.073*** (0.018) | −0.104*** (0.018) | 0.045** (0.017) | −0.021 (0.018) | 0.009 (0.017) | 0.002 (0.017) |
| Observations | 3,035 | | | | | 3,073 | | | | |

*** $p<0.001$, ** $p<0.01$, * $p<0.05$.
*Note*: Probabilities of agreement with standard errors in parentheses.

Chapter 4

# Public Priorities During a Pandemic: Cross-national Comparisons

*C. Cozette Comer*

*Virginia Tech, USA*

### Abstract

This chapter explores the financial aspects of resolving the COVID-19 pandemic, including respondents' feelings about their country going into more debt and perceptions of how public funding should be spent. A factor analysis reveals spending priorities could be classified into three broad areas: Welfare (e.g., funding social welfare and research), Development (e.g., business, infrastructure, and international development), and Security (e.g., police and military). Finnish residents were more likely to support spending on welfare while Americans were more likely to support spending on development. There was no difference between the nations for supporting spending on the security state. Importantly, confidence in institutions was negatively correlated with supporting spending on welfare but positively correlated with supporting spending in development and security. Potentially confounding factors such as having been sick with COVID-19, worrying about the pandemic, news consumption about COVID-19, social capital, life satisfaction, and feelings toward the future were included in the model to determine if these mediated or moderated the relationship between confidence in institutions and support for various types of spending. While none of the variables mediated the relationship between confidence and spending priorities, worrying about COVID-19, social isolation, and social capital were related to increased support for spending on welfare, while being sick with COVID-19 and social capital were related to increased support for spending on the security state. The analyses reveal that pandemic-related factors influence spending priorities, but these did

---

*Perceptions of a Pandemic: A Cross-Continental Comparison of Citizen Perceptions, Attitudes, and Behaviors During COVID-19, 49–61*
Copyright © 2025 by C. Cozette Comer
Published under exclusive licence by Emerald Publishing Limited
doi:10.1108/978-1-83608-624-620241004

## 50  C. Cozette Comer

not overcome the influence of demographic factors and the general level of confidence one had in the institutions of society.

*Keywords*: Spending priorities; national debt and COVID-19 mitigation strategies; public spending; defense spending; taxation and COVID-19

## Introduction

The allocation of public spending to mitigate and ideally quash the negative effects of a pandemic is an important consideration. The distribution of public funds in a democratic society should, at least in part, be informed by public opinion. In this chapter, we explore the differences and similarities between the public's thoughts about how state funds should be spent during the first year of the COVID-19 pandemic in the United States and Finland.

## The Cross-national Context of COVID-19

As noted in Chapter 1, one of the key distinctions between these countries is that the US culture is market-driven, while Finland is a more state-oriented society (see Alesina & Glaeser, 2006; Gilbert, 2004; Greve, 2007; Hass, 2006; Lin, 2004; Räsänen, 2006). Given this, we would predict that Finns would be more likely than Americans to support state spending to address the COVID-19 crisis. In addition, Finland's debt-to-GDP ratio was almost half the United States' ratio in 2020, which would suggest more room for increasing governmental spending. While Finland's debt-to-GDP ratio was 60.2% in 2020, the United States' was a staggering 110.1% (International Monetary Fund (IMF), 2023). Finally, the political parties leading each country in the initial stages of the pandemic would suggest Finland would be more favorable toward using state funds for combatting the pandemic. In Finland, Prime Minister Marin's Social Democratic Party has historically favored deficit spending, while President Trump's Republican Party has traditionally been opposed to government spending, at least rhetorically. These factors suggest that Finns would be likely to support government spending to combat the pandemic more so than their American counterparts.

## Willingness to Increasing National Debt

Aligned with our predictions, most Finnish respondents (nearly 40%) agreed that it would be okay to raise the national debt to address the COVID-19 pandemic (see Fig. 4.1). US respondents, on the other hand, had similar rates of responding in agreement or feeling neutral about increasing national debt in response to the pandemic (at approximately 30.8% and 30%, respectively). Likewise, more US than Finnish respondents disagreed or strongly disagreed with the idea of increasing national debt to handle the pandemic. Nearly the same proportion (approximately 15%) of Finnish and US respondents, respectively, strongly agreed with raising debt to respond to COVID-19.

Public Priorities During a Pandemic 51

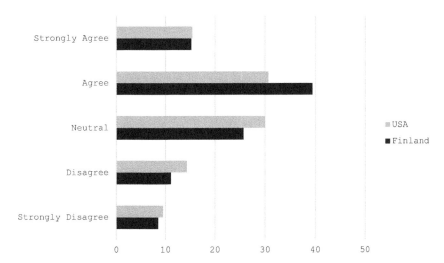

Fig. 4.1. Percent of Respondents Willing to Increase National Debt to Address COVID-19.

However, in addition to the more state-centric approaches of Finns relative to Americans, it is important to consider the two nations' relative fiscal health for absorbing additional debt. While Finland is known to be a far more generous state and more supportive of state interventions than the United States, there has been mounting concern in Finland over continuing these spending policies (Kauranen, 2023). Yet, the American public is also well known to be unsupportive of governmental programs, especially those delivered by direct government spending (see Faricy & Ellis, 2014; Gilbert, 2004).

Generally, a lower debt-to-GDP ratio is ideal, as it signals a country is producing more than it owes, placing it on a strong financial footing. Concerns about the state's ability to repay its debt increase as the debt-to-GDP ratio increases, and debt-to-GDP ratios exceeding 77% for prolonged periods are associated with significant slowdowns in economic growth (Grennes et al., 2013). Even excluding intragovernmental debt, the debt held by the public in the United States was $16.8 trillion at the end of 2019, which was equal to 79% of GDP (Congressional Budget Office, 2023). Considering that the federal government's debt increased at a faster rate between 2009 and 2019 than at any time since World War II and reached its highest levels since immediately after that war (Congressional Budget Office, 2023), the American public would likely be hesitant to add to this debt. By contrast, in 2019, EDP debt held by the government of Finland was €155.6 million or 64.9% of their GDP (Statistics Finland, 2022). The Finnish population may feel less pressure to lower the debt ratio than their US counterparts.

Given these conditions, we anticipate that Americans would likely embrace more market-oriented priorities during the pandemic while Finns would be more likely to support state-oriented priorities. Therefore, when it comes to how money should be spent during the COVID-19 pandemic, we expect Finnish respondents to be favorable of state-oriented spending and US respondents to be more favorable of market spending.

## How Government Funding Should Be Allocated in Response to the Pandemic

To investigate priorities in public spending, we asked US and Finnish citizens questions about if they thought certain types of funding should be modified during the COVID-19 pandemic. When it comes to how respondents want to spend public funding during COVID-19, we used factor analysis to identify three areas: welfare, development, and security. "Welfare" spending includes funding allocated to (1) the public sector, (2) public healthcare, (3) universities, (4) scientific research, (5) public schools, (6) pensions, and (7) social benefits. "Development" spending includes funding to support (1) businesses, (2) transportation, (3) immigration, (4) development aid, (5) culture, and (6) environmental protection. Finally, the "security" spending category is comprised of (1) military and (2) police. How we assigned different spending areas to a grouping is discussed in the Appendix.

Basic frequencies (see Fig. 4.2) indicate that most respondents from both countries preferred to maintain, rather than increase or decrease spending across all three categories. Of all respondents, most wanted to reduce development-related spending and increase welfare-related spending, more than other categories, respectively. Unsurprisingly, within the welfare category, Finnish respondents were more supportive of spending on public health and universities compared to US respondents. Within the security category, support for increasing police funding was higher in Finland than the United States. Although the majority of Americans have historically expressed good relations with the police, the 2020 Black Lives Matter protests sparked questions regarding police funding with the mantra of defunding the police (see Wright et al., 2023). This likely contributed to the lack of support among Americans for increasing police funding among respondents in this survey (see Novick & Pickett, 2022, for a discussion).

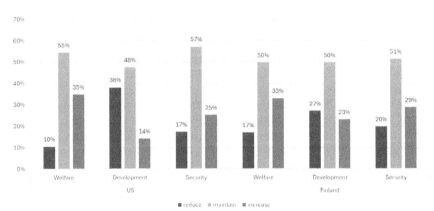

Fig. 4.2. Percent of Respondents Wanting to Reduce, Maintain, or Increase Each Spending Category by Country.

## Support for Welfare, Development, and Security Spending

Moving to a multivariate analysis (see Table 4.1), we regress support for the three types of spending on several factors using data from the United States and Finland in April 2020. Our major variables of interest are country and confidence in those running major institutions. To measure confidence in institutions, we factor analyze respondent's expressed levels of confidence in people running the following entities: (1) banks, (2) major companies, (3) organized religion, (4) education, (5) executive government, (6) organized labor, (7) press, (8) medicine, (9) media, (10) legal system, (11) science, (12) the legislative government, and (13) military. Ultimately, these groups were combined into three categories: institutions, press, and science. "Institutions" reflects confidence in those running banks, major companies, organized religion, the executive government, organized labor, the legal system, the legislative government, and the military. "Press" was comprised of being confident in those who run the press and the media. Finally, "science" reflects having confidence in those who run education, medicine, and science.

As controlling for potentially confounding factors allows for a more precise understanding of how respondents preferred to spend national funds during the COVID-19 pandemic, we also include several control variables. The models predicting support for welfare spending, development spending, and security spending include country and our measures of confidence in institutions, confidence in the press, confidence in science, social capital, media consumption, satisfaction with life, feelings of isolation, beliefs about future prospects, age, sex, education, support for the political party in power, immigrant status, race, worry about COVID-19, and being sick from COVID-19.

Unsurprisingly, US respondents were less likely than Finnish respondents to want to increase spending on welfare-related areas like public schools, healthcare, pensions, and so on. This is to be expected given the anti-statist nature of the United States. US respondents were more likely than Finnish respondents to spend public funds on development-related areas such as supporting businesses, transportation infrastructure, and culture & art. There was no statistical difference between countries in terms of spending on security.

Confidence in major institutions was negatively correlated with wanting to spend on welfare. In other words, those who trust institutions like banks, companies, organized religion, or military are less likely to support spending public funds on welfare-related areas like public schools or healthcare. In contrast, confidence in these institutions was positively correlated with spending in development (e.g., support for business, arts & culture, and environmental protection) and security (military or police). Confidence in press was positively correlated with spending in both the welfare and development categories but negatively correlated with spending in security-related areas. Interestingly, there is a statistically significant positive association between confidence in science (or medicine) and spending on welfare, yet the relationship is not statistically significant in either the development or security model.

Social capital, or respondents' feelings of connection to society, was positively correlated with both spending on welfare and security. Correlation with welfare

Table 4.1.   Factors Predicting Public Spending Priorities in Finland and the United States: Welfare Spending, Development Spending, and Security Spending.

| | Welfare Spending | | Development Spending | | Security Spending | |
|---|---|---|---|---|---|---|
| | **Estimate** | **Std Error** | **Estimate** | **Std Error** | **Estimate** | **Std Error** |
| The United States | −0.494*** | 0.036 | 0.449*** | 0.035 | −0.094** | 0.038 |
| Age | 0.004*** | 0.001 | −0.010*** | 0.001 | 0.010*** | 0.001 |
| Female | 0.130*** | 0.031 | 0.026 | 0.030 | 0.034 | 0.033 |
| College degree | −0.135*** | 0.032 | 0.057* | 0.031 | −0.115*** | 0.034 |
| Support party in Power | −0.011 | 0.034 | 0.018 | 0.033 | 0.016 | 0.036 |
| Immigrant | 0.024 | 0.066 | −0.054 | 0.064 | 0.010 | 0.069 |
| White | −0.014 | 0.054 | −0.140*** | 0.052 | 0.017 | 0.056 |
| Worry about COVID-19 | 0.182*** | 0.028 | 0.017 | 0.027 | −0.022 | 0.029 |
| Sick from COVID-19 | −0.002 | 0.038 | −0.044 | 0.037 | 0.097** | 0.040 |
| Total media consumption | 0.036** | 0.018 | −0.037** | 0.018 | 0.029 | 0.019 |
| Social capital | 0.014*** | 0.004 | 0.006 | 0.004 | 0.010** | 0.005 |
| Isolated | 0.021** | 0.009 | 0.033*** | 0.009 | 0.006 | 0.010 |
| Life satisfaction | −0.007 | 0.009 | 0.005 | 0.009 | −0.004 | 0.010 |
| Future prospects | −0.011 | 0.009 | 0.013 | 0.009 | 0.014 | 0.009 |
| Confidence in institutions | −0.126*** | 0.018 | 0.104*** | 0.017 | 0.378*** | 0.019 |
| Confidence in press | 0.125*** | 0.017 | 0.352*** | 0.016 | −0.130*** | 0.018 |
| Confidence in science | 0.347*** | 0.017 | 0.022 | 0.016 | −0.007 | 0.017 |

*** $p < 0.001$ ** $p < 0.01$ * $p < 0.05$.

*Note*: Adj $R^2$s range from 0.18 to 0.29.

*Public Priorities During a Pandemic*    55

makes sense, as one is more likely to want to support others if they feel connected to others in their community. Similarly, the desire to protect the community, or support spending in security-related activities (e.g., law enforcement and national defense) may be driven in part by a desire to protect those in their community. Interestingly, feelings of isolation were also positively correlated with support for spending in welfare- and development-related initiatives. Although high social capital is correlated with welfare spending, isolation may lead to a desire for more support from the community through welfare-related spending. Development, which includes spending on areas such as transportation and immigration, may also be correlated by the desire for more connection with the community among those who are otherwise feeling isolated.

Overall media consumption was positively correlated with spending on welfare-related project and negatively correlated with spending on development-related project. This may be due, at least in part, to how these spending categories were framed by the media respondents were consuming. It is likely that commonly consumed media spoke of institutions directly related to the pandemic positively, at least for the most part. For example, the welfare category contains items like scientific research and public health, both of which would be directly related to the mitigation of negative pandemic-related outcomes. These findings comport with research presented in Chapter 5 of this book by Koivula and Martilla that identified that media omnivores are more likely to trust in experts, which would also explain a willingness to support these categories of spending. In contrast, the development category includes areas like businesses, transportation, and culture which could only tangentially be related to the pandemic and likely framed by media neutrally or in a manner unrelated to the pandemic. This category also includes items like immigration and environmental protection which have been politicized in media, both in the United States and in Finland.

Respondents who were worried about COVID-19 were more likely to support spending in welfare. It seems reasonable that those more concerned with the present pandemic would be more supportive of spending in areas directly related to activities that could mitigate harm caused by the pandemic, such as scientific research, healthcare, and social benefits. Having been sick with COVID-19, however, was only statistically significantly correlated with spending in security-related activities. Perhaps the experience of having the illness creates a higher sense of urgency that, in turn, leads to more support for spending on force-based mitigation tactics.

Finally, wishing to increase spending in welfare was more likely among females and those without a college degree. While those without a college degree were also more likely to support security-related spending, those with a college degree were more likely to support spending on development (but only with significance of $p<0.1$). Race was only statistically significant in the development model, suggesting white respondents are less likely to support development-related spending. Age was a statistically significant factor for all three spending areas; positively correlated with welfare and security, but negatively correlated with development. This relationship makes sense considering risk tolerance lowers with age

## 56 C. Cozette Comer

(Albert & Duffy, 2012). This desire for consistency makes sense especially during exceptionally uncertain times such as those of a pandemic, which is particularly dangerous for elderly populations.

## Spending Is Vital and Confidence in Institutions Is Necessary for Public Support

As expected, respondents from Finland were overall more supportive of spending compared to respondents from the United States. This is especially true for spending within the welfare category – and even more so when it comes to spending on universities and public health. Contrastingly, respondents from the United States were more supportive than those from Finland of spending in development-related areas. This is somewhat aligned with our expectations that market-oriented priorities would be preferable to those from the United States. However, the development category also included immigration, development aid, environmental protection, transportation, and culture, which do not necessarily translate to support for spending toward private, rather than public solutions.

Confidence in the press and confidence in institutions were each associated with the desire to spend more in development-related initiatives; likewise, confidence in science was positively correlated with wanting to spend more on welfare-related initiatives. Interestingly, confidence in institutions was also associated with a lack of support for welfare-related spending. We now know that government-funded research and collaborative efforts between private and public entities (Druedahl et al., 2021) resulted in vaccines that saved lives (Agrawal et al., 2023) and accelerated the end of the pandemic. In other words, spending in both private and public sectors was vital for ending the pandemic; yet, support for such spending depends upon the public's confidence in these institutions. This fact may be concerning as, according to Lupia et al. (2024), confidence in institutions writ large has declined over time in the United States. Indeed, based on Gallup data that track confidence in institutions, Americans' confidence in major US institutions reached all-time lows in the early 2020s (see Jones, 2022). Most strikingly, only 7% of Americans said they had a great deal or quite a lot of confidence in the US congress in 2022 (Jones, 2022). In Finland, public trust in institutions remains high, particularly trust in government institutions and the police (OECD, 2020, 2021), but evidence suggests this trust is slowly eroding. For example, the percentage of Finns reporting that they trusted their government decreased from 76% in 2007 to 64% in 2019 (OECD, 2021). While this is still comparatively high levels of trust, it nevertheless reflects a disturbing trend. These trends of lower levels of trust in civic institutions across both the United States and Finland do not bode well for generating support for additional spending should some future crises require it.

Likewise, the negative relationship between confidence in institutions and spending in welfare indicates that the problem of gaining support for vital spending is not as simple as increasing confidence in institutions across the board. Based on our data, confidence in major institutions increased support for developmental and security measures but not for welfare approaches. It is somewhat

*Public Priorities During a Pandemic* **57**

alarming that increasing confidence in central institutions reduces support for spending on welfare approaches since it was spending on public health measures and scientific research that most contributed to the discovery of a vaccine and the eventual ending of the pandemic – which are key factors in the welfare approach. Given this, increasing confidence in central institutions may inadvertently lead to pursuing less efficacious policies.

Building trust in science should be an ongoing endeavor. Some barriers to instilling confidence in scientific institutions may be simple misinformation about how funding is already allocated. For example, Goldfarb and Kriner (2017) found many Americans overestimated how much federal money was already designated for scientific research. But, if provided with accurate information about federal spending, respondents were more likely to support an increase in government spending on scientific research.

Science itself has also been politicized and undermined with mis- and disinformation, which contributes to the reduction in trust and confidence in relevant institutions. Recommendations for mitigating these kinds of harms tend toward social interventions such as education (e.g., Sheng et al., 2021; Shu et al., 2020) and strategic communication through approaches such as storytelling and emotional appeals (e.g., Goldstein et al., 2020). Especially with social media, getting ahead of bad information online using machine learning and other algorithmic approaches (e.g., Shu et al., 2020) should also be considered. In any case, it is important to build and maintain trust in scientific institutions before these institutions need more resources. In the United States, invested persons may specifically want to target conservatives as their trust in science has declined since the 1970s, illustrating a concerning trend well before the COVID-19 pandemic (Gauchat, 2012).

While there were no substantial differences in support for funding security-related initiatives between the United States and Finland, Finnish respondents were more supportive of funding law enforcement at the disaggregate level. Again, confidence in these institutions is important and those with confidence in institutions were associated with desire to spend on police and military. Social capital was also positively correlated with desire to spend on security-related initiatives. The dip in support for law enforcement spending among US respondents is likely related to the 2020 Black Lives Matter movement that both highlighted existing poor public confidence in and directly encouraged defunding of police-related institutions.

During the COVID-19 pandemic, spending in security-related areas did not appear as vital for mitigating related harms as spending in development and welfare areas. For example, the military only played a minor role in the development of the vaccine (Druedahl et al., 2021). Law enforcement was employed to uphold other mitigation tactics such as enforcing curfews, social distancing, and shelter-in-place orders (International Association of Chiefs of Police, 2020). However, encouraging compliance through police would only be useful in societies with preexisting collaborative relationships with law enforcement. In fact, attempting to enforce pandemic-related regulation without first establishing public confidence and trust in police can potentially be counterproductive. Relying

**58** *C. Cozette Comer*

on law enforcement in communities with low levels of trust in the policing institution would be at best unhelpful and potentially result in even less compliance. Research clearly demonstrates that citizens comply with police orders when those citizens' perceptions of police legitimacy are high (Bradford et al., 2021; Hawdon, 2008; Mazerolle et al., 2013; Pryce & Gainey, 2022; Reisig & Trinkner, 2024). In cases where perceived legitimacy is low, any attempt by the police to force compliance can result in resentment and greater non-compliance (Hawdon, 2008). Recent evidence from Australia shows this general finding applies to COVID-19 mandates (McCarthy et al., 2021). Therefore, relying on police to promote compliance with health-protective mandates can work, but they are likely to only be effective when police–community relations are positive.

Yet, it is difficult for other institutions to enforce mandates since they lack the authority to do so outside their narrow scope. For example, a business can enforce a mask mandate, but they can do so only when a person is physically in their business. And, of course, there is a built-in disincentive for businesses to enforce mandates since they run the risk of alienating potential customers by doing so. Only the police have the authority to enforce laws widely. As such, it is important to understand when doing so is effective. As noted above, this would likely be effective only in cases where the police already enjoy a positive relationship with the community. Such a positive relationship between the police and community members is more evident in Finland than in the United States. While the police enjoy widespread support in both Finland and the United States, Finnish police enjoy some of the highest levels of perceived legitimacy in the world (e.g., Laird & Charman, 2023; Lehtonen & De Carlo, 2019; Kääriäinen & Sirén, 2011; Vuorensyrjä & Rauta, 2020). For example, in a study of European nations, Finland trailed only Denmark in trust in police procedural fairness with well over 80% of the population reporting high levels of trust (see Jackson et al., 2014). By comparison, there is a large gap in terms of police legitimacy between white Americans, Hispanic Americans, and Black Americans (see Brown & Lloyd, 2023). Although support for the Finnish police is beginning to erode among minorities and immigrant groups (see Egharevba, 2021; Vuorensyrjä & Rauta, 2020), support for the police is higher in Finland than in the United States. This implies that Finland may be in a better position to rely on the police to compel compliance than the United States.

However, evidence suggests that with a careful, theoretically informed approach, police can improve their relationships with communities that have historically not trusted them and by doing so elevate citizen perceptions of police legitimacy (see Hawdon, 2008; Hawdon et al., 2003). Moreover, citizens are more responsive to the police if they work with community organizations that have a history of working with the police (Hawdon & Ryan, 2011). The police could rely on parochialism that operates through organizations instead of directly, as this style of community engagement appears to be effective even in areas with low levels of trust in police and social capital (see Carr, 2003). Therefore, it is theoretically possible for the government to have police and other security officers' partner with community groups to help promote compliance with health-protective mandates.

Low confidence and trust in the institutions that are vital to mitigation of harm during and recovery from a global pandemic is concerning as our analysis indicates trust is highly associated with willingness to spend public funds. Trust, and by extension confidence, in institutions can be built through transparency, communication, integrity, reliability, and fairness (OECD, 2021). Those countries with high levels of trust and confidence in their public institutions, like Finland, should work to maintain that trust. Countries like the United States need to work toward building that trust before trust in core institutions is necessary to reduce harm from a public calamity.

## Conclusion

Although our analysis did not demonstrate any meaningful difference between US and Finnish respondents' willingness to increase national debt in response to COVID-19, we did find US respondents were less likely than Finnish respondents to support welfare-related spending increases and more likely to support development-related spending. Spending in both public and private sectors is vital for addressing global catastrophes like the COVID-19 pandemic and, in democratic societies, it is important that the public supports that spending. In both the United States and Finland, our analysis indicates support for spending in a category (e.g., welfare) is associated with confidence in related institutions. The exception, however, being higher levels of confidence in institutions like banks, major companies, organized religion, the executive government, organized labor, the legal system, the legislative government, and the military were negatively associated with support for spending in welfare-related areas such as the public sector, public healthcare, universities, scientific research, public schools, pensions, and social benefits. Therefore, efforts to increase confidence in institutions as a means of increasing support for relevant spending should be targeted and more nuanced analyses should be conducted. Whether for scientific research institutions – public and private – that can aid in the development of vaccines or police entities that have the unique authority to enforce mitigation strategies, it is vital to establish confidence prior to the next pandemic.

## References

Agrawal, V., Sood, N., & Whaley, C. (2023). *The impact of the global COVID-19 vaccination campaign on all-cause mortality (w31812; p. w31812)*. National Bureau of Economic Research. https://doi.org/10.3386/w31812

Albert, S. M., & Duffy, J. (2012). Differences in risk aversion between young and older adults. *Neuroscience and Neuroeconomics, 1,* 3–9.

Alesina, A., & Glaeser, E. L. (2006). Why are welfare states in the US and Europe so different?. *Horizons Stratégiques, 2*(2), 51–61.

Bradford, B., Jackson, J., & Milani, J. (2021). Police legitimacy. *The Encyclopedia of Research Methods in Criminology and Criminal Justice, 2,* 642–650.

Brown, M. C., III, & Lloyd, C. (2023). *Black Americans less confident, satisfied with local police*. Gallup. https://news.gallup.com/poll/511064/black-americans-less-confident-satisfied-local-police.aspx#:~:text=About%20seven%20in%2010%20U.S.,and%20Hispanic%20Americans%20(64%25)

## 60 C. Cozette Comer

Carr, P. J. (2003). The new parochialism: The implications of the Beltway case for arguments concerning informal social control. *American Journal of Sociology*, *108*(6), 1249–1291.

Congressional Budget Office. (2020). Federal debt: A primer. https://www.cbo.gov/publication/56309

Druedahl, L. C., Minssen, T., & Price, W. N. (2021). Collaboration in times of crisis: A study on COVID-19 vaccine R&D partnerships. *Vaccine*, *39*(42), 6291–6295. https://doi.org/10.1016/j.vaccine.2021.08.101

Egharevba, S. (2021). Tenuous relations: Ethnic–racial cultural and police disrespect in Finland. *International Journal of Police Science & Management*, *23*(2), 133–144.

Faricy, C., & Ellis, C. (2014). Public attitudes toward social spending in the United States: The differences between direct spending and tax expenditures. *Political Behavior*, *36*(1), 53–76. https://doi.org/10.1007/s11109-013-9225-5

Gauchat, G. (2012). Politicization of science in the public sphere: A study of public trust in the United States, 1974 to 2010. *American Sociological Review*, *77*(2), 167–187.

Gilbert, G. (2004). Is Europe living up to its obligations to refugees? *European Journal of International Law*, *15*(5), 963–987. https://doi.org/10.1093/ejil/15.5.963

Goldfarb, J. L., & Kriner, D. L. (2017). Building public support for science spending: Misinformation, motivated reasoning, and the power of corrections. *Science Communication*, *39*(1), 77–100. https://doi.org/10.1177/1075547016688325

Goldstein, C. M., Murray, E. J., Beard, J., Schnoes, A. M., & Wang, M. L. (2020). Science communication in the age of misinformation. *Annals of Behavioral Medicine*, *54*(12), 985–990. https://doi.org/10.1093/abm/kaaa088

Greve, B. (2007). What characterise the Nordic welfare state model. *Journal of Social Sciences*, *3*(2), 43–51.

Hass, J. (2006). Economic sociology: An introduction. Routledge.

Hawdon, J. (2008). Legitimacy, trust, social capital, and policing styles: A theoretical statement. *Police Quarterly*, *11*(2), 182–201.

Hawdon, J., & Ryan, J. (2011). Neighborhood organizations and resident assistance to police. *Sociological Forum*, *26*(4), 897–920.

Hawdon, J. E., Ryan, J., & Griffin, S. P. (2003). Policing tactics and perceptions of police legitimacy. *Police Quarterly*, *6*(4), 469–491.

International Monetary Fund (IMF). (2023). *Annual report 2023*. https://www.imf.org/external/pubs/ft/ar/2023/english/

International Association of Chiefs of Police. (2020). *Law enforcement and COVID-19*. U.S. Department of Justice, Community Oriented Policing Services. https://portal.cops.usdoj.gov/resourcecenter?item=cops-w0905

Jackson, J., Kuha, J., Hough, M., Bradford, B., Hohl, K., & Gerber, M. M. (2014). *Trust and legitimacy across Europe: A FIDUCIA report on comparative public attitudes towards legal authority*. Available at SSRN 2272975

Jones, J. (2022). *Confidence in U.S. institutions down; average at new low*. Gallup. https://news.gallup.com/poll/394283/confidence-institutions-down-average-new-low.aspx

Kääriäinen, J., & Sirén, R. (2011). Trust in the police, generalized trust and reporting crime. European Journal of Criminology, *8*(1), 65–81.

Kauranen, S. A. (2023). Finland·FDI screening overview: A notable increase in scrutiny. *European Competition & Regulatory Law Review*, *7*(3), 169–173. https://doi.org/10.21552/core/2023/3/7

Laird, A., & Charman, S. (2023). 'Accidental' procedural justice: The Finnish approach to policing. *International Journal of Police Science & Management*, *25*(1), 17–29.

Lehtonen, M., & De Carlo, L. (2019). Diffuse institutional trust and specific institutional mistrust in Nordic participatory planning: Experience from contested urban projects. *Planning Theory and Practice*, *20*(2), 203–220.

# Public Priorities During a Pandemic 61

Lin, K. (2004). Sectors, agents and rationale: A study of the Scandinavian welfare states with special reference to the welfare society model. *Acta Sociologica, 47*(2), 141–157. https://doi.org/10.1177/0001699304043852

Lupia, A., Allison, D. B., Jamieson, K. H., Heimberg, J., Skipper, M., & Wolf, S. M. (2024). Trends in U.S. public confidence in science and opportunities for progress. *Proceedings of the National Academy of Sciences, 121*(11), e2319488121.

Mazerolle, L., Bennett, S., Davis, J., Sargeant, E., & Manning, M. (2013). Procedural justice and police legitimacy: A systematic review of the research evidence. *Journal of Experimental Criminology, 9*, 245–274.

McCarthy, M., Murphy, K., Sargeant, E., & Williamson, H. (2021). Policing COVID-19 physical distancing measures: Managing defiance and fostering compliance among individuals least likely to comply. *Policing and Society, 31*(5), 601–620.

Novick, R., & Pickett, J. T. (2022). Black Lives Matter, protest policing, and voter support for police reform in Portland, Oregon. *Race and Justice, 14*(3), 368–392. https://doi.org/10.1177/21533687221117281.

OECD. (2020). *OECD economic surveys: Finland 2020.* OECD Publishing. https://dx.doi.org/10.1787/673aeb7f-en

OECD. (2021). *Drivers of trust in public institutions in Finland.* OECD. https://doi.org/10.1787/52600c9e-en

Pryce, D. K., & Gainey, R. (2022). Race differences in public satisfaction with and trust in the local police in the context of George Floyd protests: An analysis of residents' experiences and attitudes. *Criminal Justice Studies, 35*(1), 74–92.

Räsänen, P. (2006). Consumption disparities in information society: Comparing the traditional and digital divides in Finland. *International Journal of Sociology and Social Policy, 26*(1/2), 48–62. https://doi.org/10.1108/01443330610644425

Reisig, M. D., & Trinkner, R. (2024). Distinguishing between normative and non-normative motivations to obey the police: Furthering the development of a police legitimacy scale. *Policing: An International Journal, 47*(1), 50–65.

Sheng, A. Y., Gottlieb, M., & Welsh, L. (2021). Leveraging learner-centered educational frameworks to combat health mis/disinformation. *AEM Education and Training, 5*(4), e10711. https://doi.org/10.1002/aet2.10711

Shu, K., Bhattacharjee, A., Alatawi, F., Nazer, T. H., Ding, K., Karami, M., & Liu, H. (2020). Combating disinformation in a social media age. *WIREs Data Mining and Knowledge Discovery, 10*(6), e1385. https://doi.org/10.1002/widm.1385

Statistics Finland. (2022). *General government EDP deficit and debt, annually, 1975–2022.* Statistics Finland. https://pxdata.stat.fi/PxWeb/pxweb/en/StatFin/StatFin__jali/statfin_jali_pxt_122g.px/table/tableViewLayout1/

Vuorensyrjä, M., & Rauta, J. (2020). *Police barometer 2020: Citizens' assessments of police activities and the state of Finland's internal security.* Ministry of the Interior Publications (No. 2020/12). http://urn.fi/URN:ISBN:978-952-324-641-6

Wright, J. E., Gaozhao, D., Dukes, K., & Templeton, D. S. (2023). The power of protest on policing: Black Lives Matter protest and civilian evaluation of the police. *Public Administration Review, 83*(1), 130–143.

Section 2

# Media as a Complicating Factor

Chapter 5

# Trust in Experts According to Media Consumption and Government Satisfaction in the United States and Finland

*Aki Koivula, Eetu Marttila and Pekka Räsänen*

*University of Turku, Finland*

## Abstract

This chapter examines the relationship between media consumption during COVID-19 and its effect on trust in experts. Successful crisis management requires risk assessment and rapid decisions, and decision-making in the crisis is often based on multidimensional and conflicting information, which highlights the importance of trust. Here, the aim is to examine how daily media consumption is associated with trust in experts and satisfaction with government response during the pandemic. Media consumption was defined by how many different media platforms respondents used daily, grouped into three broad categories: (1) broadcast media, including television and radio; (2) journalistic media, including newspapers and periodicals; and (3) social media, including social network sites and discussion forums. The results of the analyses show that trust in experts strengthened as the crisis progressed, but satisfaction with the government declined. Omnivorous media consumption – those who consumed several different forms of media – increased trust in experts as well as satisfaction with the government. Particularly, one-sided and social media-based media consumption was related to declined trust. That is, those who used only one form of media and those who relied heavily on social media alone expressed lower levels of trust in experts. The mediation analysis showed that the association between media consumption and government satisfaction was partly indirect through trust in experts.

---

Perceptions of a Pandemic: A Cross-Continental Comparison of Citizen Perceptions, Attitudes, and Behaviors During COVID-19, 65–83
Copyright © 2025 by Aki Koivula, Eetu Marttila, and Pekka Räsänen
Published under exclusive licence by Emerald Publishing Limited
doi:10.1108/978-1-83608-624-620241005

## 66  *Aki Koivula et al.*

Overall, the study reinforces the importance of media as a moderator of messages during crisis management.

*Keywords*: Media consumption; political trust; longitudinal research; crisis messaging; COVID-19

## Introduction

Successful crisis management requires risk assessment and rapid decisions (Slovic & Weber, 2002). The decision-making in the crisis is often based on multidimensional and conflicting information, which highlights the importance of trust (e.g., Luhmann, 1979). Current studies have shown that trust is an important predictor of successful public health policy implementation during the COVID-19 outbreak (Bollyky et al., 2022; Oksanen et al., 2020). Also, research has pointed out that trust is associated with vaccination intentions (e.g., Wynen et al., 2022) and compliance with protective measures (e.g., Kestilä-Kekkonen et al., 2022; Plohl & Musil, 2021). However, most previous studies have focused on generalized institutional or political trust, not specifying which authorities, politicians, or people are trusted. In particular, the extent to which trust in experts varies during a pandemic and what factors explain its variation as the pandemic progresses remains an open question.

Trust in social relations arises primarily from three sources: past experiences, future expectations, and social networks (Schilke et al., 2021). When individuals evaluate their trust in experts, they assess their past performance and weigh their trust based on how experts have met their expectations in the past. Another way to determine individuals' trust in experts is by looking at how much they value their relationship with the expert, as trust is built when a person evaluates the expert's reliability over time and decides to continue the relationship based on that assessment. Also, trust in experts is created in a broader social context and varies according to the extent to which the "object of trust" is embedded in citizens' wider social networks (Coleman, 1988; Granovetter, 1985). In this study, we approach trust to experts from a network perspective and assume that individuals' level of trust in experts depends on the information that is transmitted through indirect links between different actors and citizens.

We focus on two distinct perspectives when examining predictors of trusting in experts. First, we assume that citizens' trust in experts is linked to their ideological views and political beliefs. For example, it is possible that politicians do not share the views of experts and transmit information that suits their own agenda and partisan consideration, thus reducing the credibility of experts (Ban et al., 2022). From previous studies, we also know that citizens tend to follow leaders in the initial stages of the crisis (Baker & Oneal, 2001) and that political leaders influence citizens' attitudes and beliefs in general (Druckman et al., 2013). Thus, it is possible that citizens' perceptions of politicians may also be reflected in their trust in experts in the crisis. Second, we assume that citizens' trust in experts is affected by their media consumption habits. In general, individuals' attitudes toward science and technology are influenced by the types of traditional media channels they use (Nisbet et al., 2002).

However, today's media environments are diverse, expanded, and fragmented, and citizens can search for information from multiple sources and connect directly with experts, authorities, and decision-makers (Chadwick, 2017). Various platforms – such as social networking sites and discussion forums – allow citizens to participate in discussions and policy debates on the infection rate of the pandemic, together with experts, public authorities, and the media. Accordingly, social media plays a potentially key role in expert trust, with an increasing flow of alternative crisis information without explicit moderation (Mihelj et al., 2022). Given that scoping studies have indicated a wide range of inaccurate information displayed on these various channels (Vos, 2021), the media have potentially a considerable influence on shaping trust in experts.

In this study, we examine *how Finns and Americans trusted on medical and epidemiological experts to find solutions to manage the pandemic*. First, we analyze whether satisfaction with national government explains trust in experts solving the crisis in the United States and Finland. Second, we consider media consumption to be the key factor contributing to the levels of trust. We examine whether different media use patterns explain trust in experts similarly across the counties. Moreover, we expect to find both cross-national and temporal differences in the levels of trust observed.

Before going to the empirical study, we define the main concepts of the study, review the previous literature, and discuss the expected difference between the United States and Finland. After this, we present the study design and describe the statistical methods used. We then present the results, which are finally discussed in relation to the previous literature.

## Literature Review

### Trust in Experts During Crisis

According to Niklas Luhmann (1979), trust is a basic element and an essential lubricant of social interaction to manage complexities of social world. Trust promotes the emergence and maintenance of cooperation and, in this respect, is essential for the social order (Balliet & Van Lange, 2013; Macy & Skvoretz, 1998). As a concept, trust refers to the tendency of a subject (A) to believe that an object (B), which can be a person, a group, or an institution, will perform as expected in a matter at hand (X) (Citrin & Stoker, 2018; PytlikZillig & Kimbrough, 2016). In other words, the essence of trust consists of the interaction between A and B in relation to X, which embodies A's expectations of B's performance, that is, whether B will meet A's expectations.

Trust is closely linked to the concepts of risk and uncertainty and is therefore critical to the construction of social relationships in times of crisis. Without the possibility of some uncertainty associated with the object's actions, the subject would not need confidence that his expectations would not be met (Luhmann, 1979;

## 68 *Aki Koivula et al.*

Schilke et al., 2021). Being related to unknown outcomes, trust makes it possible to avoid having to legislate or regulate everything, and thus to avoid the need for the subject to constantly monitor the actions of the object (Robbins, 2016). Given the crisis this study focuses on, it can be argued that trust placed in experts gives them autonomy to act without constant public scrutiny.

Furthermore, trust has also become a key instrument of governance in an uncertain and complex society (Sztompka, 1999). When trusting, the subject positions him/herself as vulnerable in relation to the object, while the object gains power in relation to the subject (Rousseau et al., 1998). This imbalance between the power of the trusting subject and the power of the trusted object is particularly relevant when considering citizens' trust in institutions such as politicians or experts. In times of crisis, the power imbalance between citizens and institutions increases as people are forced to rely more on experts because they may not have the knowledge and skills to cope on their own.

By drawing on the ABI model, trust in experts is built on the extent to which citizens can trust experts' ability, benevolence, and integrity (Mayer et al., 1995). *Ability* can be seen constituted by competence, skills, or characteristics that contribute to the effectiveness of experts in the areas where citizens expect them to be specialists (Sitkin & Roth, 1993).

*Benevolence* can be understood as the extent to which citizens believe experts are doing good for citizens in general rather than just pursuing maximum profits or benefits for themselves (Schilke et al., 2021). Finally, *integrity* reflects that citizens can rely on experts to do what they have promised to do (Cairney & Wellstead, 2021). More precisely, it can also be thought of as a perception that the expert follows certain principles that are acceptable to the citizen (Mayer et al., 1995; McFall, 1987).

The extent to which citizens can rely on the abilities of experts is linked to the fact that trust is generally reciprocal in nature, which has been particularly evident in crisis situations, where citizens have been asked to comply with recommendations (Braithwaite & Makkai, 1994; Majid et al., 2021). A voluntary compliance requires mutual trust between government and citizens (Bargain & Aminjonov, 2020), but because in modern democracies policymaking if often based on scientific knowledge, trust in experts can be considered equally important to trust in government. In this process, citizens must trust that the instructions given to them are legitimate and that following them can slow down the progression of the disease. This requires trusting in the experts that provide information about the disease and policies. In a democratic society, an effective management of pandemic also requires that experts can be confident that citizens follow their recommendations. This reciprocal relationship requires that the object of the trust, in this case the expert, has sufficient ability to convince the subject, in this case citizens, that the recommendations are worthy of compliance.

However, trust in experts is not based solely on weighed judgments about the abilities of experts. In other words, trust in the abilities of experts is not necessarily based on how they have been able to demonstrate their expertise in the past, or how they can reassure citizens of their ability to demonstrate their expertise in the future. Instead, it may also be about how the object of trust is otherwise related

*Media Consumption and Government Satisfaction* **69**

to the citizen's own social networks and the information that flows through them (Coleman, 1988; Granovetter, 1985).

When considering the indirect processes that shape citizens' trust in general, the focus is on information and its transmission (e.g., Zarolia et al., 2017). In this perspective, by drawing particularly on Coleman's (1988) ideas, we assume that trust is based on what information others convey to us about the trusted actor. In other words, the information we absorb from the news, social media, friends, and acquaintances shapes our perceptions and influences our trust. In the following sections, we will focus more specifically on the indirect processes that potentially determine citizens' trust in the abilities of experts during the pandemic crisis. We pay attention to how people may be influenced by political actors and institutions to trust experts, and how media consumption patterns determine trust in experts.

### *Trust in Experts and Government Success*

We begin our analysis by examining the role of political actors and institutions in constructing trust in experts. First, government plays a key role as opinion leaders transmit a lot of information about experts – either in support or in opposition to them (Pechar et al., 2018). On the other hand, experts and political actors can also be seen as part of the same institutional system, which means that citizens' perceptions of these separate institutions can also be aligned (e.g., Miller, 2001). Trust tends to also be generalized, which means that trusting one institution predicts trusting another. From these premises, we argue that citizens' satisfaction with the government is also strongly related to their trust in experts.

In a crisis, people's trust in politicians and national administrations typically increases. Prior research identifies the rally 'round the flag phenomenon, when citizens seek national unity under the leadership of political leaders (Baum, 2002; Mueller, 1970). Various reasons have been put forward for the rally effect, such as the fact that the emotional reaction to the fear arisen in situation drives individuals to trust authorities (Hetherington & Nelson, 2003).

One aspect of the rally effect is that in a situation of uncertainty, political decision-makers automatically acquire the status of opinion leaders, which is also reinforced by the media (Baker & Oneal, 2001). Previous studies have consistently shown that citizens are sensitive to changing their opinions and behavior based on cues from political leaders (Brader et al., 2013; Druckman et al., 2013; Slothuus, 2016). This has also been demonstrated in the COVID-19 period in the United States, where public vaccination intentions were shown to be linked to the endorsement of vaccination provided by Former President Donald Trump or Current President Joe Biden (Pink et al., 2021).

The status of opinion leadership also allows politicians to reinforce their own image while downplaying the role of others in resolving the crisis. Thus, the dependence of trust between the administration and experts can also be negative, when the administration stresses a different line than the experts, then satisfaction with the administration can predict distrust of the experts. For example, previous research from the United States has shown that people often have more generous views toward the experts than toward the government, and having trust in health

## 70  Aki Koivula et al.

experts is more stable predictor of compliance with protective actions during the pandemic than trust in government (Ahluwalia et al., 2021). This suggests that trust in experts and trust in government arise from different mechanisms but on the other hand leaves open the possibility that government and its communication can play an important role in building trust in experts. We know that in the United States, the Trump administration communicated information to the outside world that was very contradictory to general expert knowledge (Mayer, 2020) and might expect that in the United States, trust in experts is negatively related to satisfaction with government.

However, the respondent's ideological viewpoint does not always predict satisfaction (or dissatisfaction) with government action in a crisis. Thus, it is also possible that a citizen will absorb information about experts from government even if it conflicts with his or her own ideological viewpoint. This can be assumed to be the case in Finland, where citizens generally have a high level of trust in experts and smaller ideological differences between supporters of government and opposition parties than in the United States. In this case, the relationship between satisfaction with government and trust in experts can be examined through the institutional theories of trust and the *generalization* of trust.

Institutional theories of trust assume that citizens' trust in institutions is based on the performance of political systems (Hetherington, 1998) and citizens' general experiences with political institutions (Levi & Stoker, 2000). For example, in country comparisons, trust in institutions has been shown to be related to state performance, especially low levels of corruption (van der Meer & Hakhverdian, 2017). Particularly in Finland, highly publicized experts can also be seen as part of the same institutional system as politicians, which is why there is likely to be a correlation between popularity and trust between these two institutions (Saarinen et al., 2020). In other words, people may judge the performance of experts based on their satisfaction with the government. Thus, based on institutional theory, we can expect that satisfaction with government performance is related to trust (e.g., Hetherington, 1998).

### Media Use and Trust in Experts

In the previous literature, media use has been recognized as a one influential factor that affects individuals' levels of trust toward each other and institutions. However, the current evidence on the relationship between media use and its association with various dimensions of trust is mixed, and it appears that the effects are dependent on media platforms used and content consumed (e.g., Klein & Robinson, 2020; Strömbäck et al., 2016).

Earlier research has noted that during a crisis media has a significant role as a modulator of trust in citizens, politicians, and experts, and the media affects how people perceive trust in other people and the level of general trust in society (e.g., Cheung & Tse, 2008; Gross et al., 2004). Again, the evidence on the exact nature of media effects on trust in crisis situation is inconsistent. For example, the use of mainstream media appears to predict greater satisfaction with government during a crisis (Laor & Lissitsa, 2022), which could be explained by the fact that

*Media Consumption and Government Satisfaction* **71**

mainstream media outlets often align their information with official government communication (Olsson & Nord, 2015). Evidence from the time of the COVID-19 pandemic is limited, but it seems that social media use might both increase and decrease levels of trust, depending on the content consumed in social networks (Laor & Lissitsa, 2022).

Similarly, earlier research on the specific relationship between media use and trust in science has returned mixed results. While there is a general agreement upon the fact that the use of different media channels affects individuals' attitudes toward science and technology (e.g., Hmielowski et al., 2014; Nisbet et al., 2002), exact mechanisms and the differences between media usage patterns are not well understood. For example, those who consume news from television report lower levels of expert trust (Dudo et al., 2011), while consumption of periodicals and newspapers predicts higher levels of trust (Anderson et al., 2012). Also, the longitudinal evidence suggests that an increase in newspaper consumption predicted an increase in trust in scientists, whereas increase in local TV news consumption negatively predicted trust in scientists (Hmielowski et al., 2014). The research on the impact of social media use on trust in experts has also returned mixed results. First, the use of social media has been found to increase trust in experts on average (Huber et al., 2019). One reason for this is that experts may appear more approachable and understandable in social media than in traditional media (Jarreau et al., 2019; Reif et al., 2020). Second, as experimental research has shown, experts in traditional media may be perceived as more trustworthy than those in social media (Reif et al., 2020). In overall, social media changes the dynamics of science communication, which may both increase and decrease trust toward the expert institutions (van Dijck & Alinejad, 2020).

The COVID-19 pandemic has been characterized by the fragmentation of information provided by different news sources. At the beginning of the COVID-19 epidemic, social media was seen as the main channel for rapidly disseminating information about the disease globally (Chan et al., 2020). Social media can have contradictory effects, as it effectively enables both the spread of misinformation and the spread of accurate information (van Dijck & Alinejad, 2020). However, at its best, social media can provide complementary and in-depth information especially in a crisis when traditional media does not have enough information (Cuello-Garcia et al., 2020). This can also strengthen people's trust in experts and raise expectations that they can deal with a crisis. This is in line with general observations on how diverse media use can lead to both trust and distrust toward institutions (Avery, 2009).

## This Study

The objective of our empirical analysis is twofold. First, we aim to provide a descriptive assessment of the evolution of Finnish and US citizens' trust in experts, satisfaction with government actions, and media consumption during the first year of the COVID-19 pandemic. Second, we seek to analyze the interrelationships between these variables in greater depth, drawing upon the potential of panel data to detect temporal variation at the individual level. Specifically, we

## 72    Aki Koivula et al.

examine how fluctuations in government satisfaction and shifts in media consumption are reflected in trust in experts.

## Participants

In this study, the requirement for participants was to have completed both the initial survey and the wave-two survey. The wave-two survey had a response rate of 51.3% in Finland and 40.9% in the United States, with a total of 767 and 613 respondents, respectively. An attrition analysis was performed to compare the characteristics of participants who completed the wave-two survey with those who dropped out, including gender, age, and education. In Finland, the wave-two survey included more male and older participants, with 48.9% being men and a mean age of 47.5 years. The dropouts had a mean age of 41.3 years and 43.6% were men. However, there was no significant difference in educational level between participants and dropouts. In the United States, the wave-two survey also included older participants, with a mean age of 48.0 years, compared to 39.9 years for dropouts. The gender distribution was similar between participants and dropouts, with approximately 47% being men. However, participants with a higher education level were more likely to complete the wave-two survey, with 58.1% having a higher education compared to 45.6% of dropouts.

## Measures

Table 5.1 shows descriptive summary of the applied variables. The main variable whose variation we examine over the two measurement points, both between and within individuals, is *trust in experts* to solve the crisis. The variable is formed on three distinct groups: researchers, doctors, and epidemiologists. For each of these groups, respondents were asked to indicate their level of trust for the group's capability to solve the crisis. The responses were then summed, and 1 represents a complete lack of trust and 10 represents complete trust (see the Appendix for more details).

As a first explanatory variable, we examine *satisfaction with the government's handling of the crisis,* which ranged from 1 to 10 (with 1 being not satisfied and 10 being very satisfied; see the Appendix for more detail). We used this original variable throughout the analyses.

The variable "daily media consumption" refers to the number of different media platforms used daily by respondents over the last month. These platforms were categorized into three types: (1) broadcast media, such as television and radio; (2) journalistic media, including newspapers and magazines; and (3) social media, encompassing social networking sites and discussion forums. Respondents initially rated their usage on a scale of 1–10 ("Not once," "Once," "More than once but not weekly," "Once a week," "Several times a week," "Once a day," "Several times a day," "Once an hour," "Several times an hour," and "All the time"). To focus on the daily consumption patterns, we constructed a binary variable by grouping options 6–10 into category 1, while the remaining options were assigned to category 0. We examined these variables both individually and

*Media Consumption and Government Satisfaction* **73**

Table 5.1. Descriptive Statistics.

| | Finland | United States | Total |
|---|---|---|---|
| *Continuous variables*: | | | |
| Trust in experts (Range 1–10) | 7.623 (1.996) | 7.420 (2.332) | 7.533 (2.153) |
| Satisfaction with government (Range 1–10) | 6.639 (2.317) | 4.993 (2.964) | 5.912 (2.746) |
| Age (Range 16–76) | 50.042 (14.208) | 53.316 (13.825) | 51.487 (14.131) |
| *Categorical variables* | | | |
| Daily media consumption | | | |
| Broadcast | | | |
| No | 254 (16.5%) | 157 (12.9%) | 411 (14.9%) |
| Yes | 1,288 (83.5%) | 1,061 (87.1%) | 2,349 (85.1%) |
| Print | | | |
| No | 221 (14.3%) | 468 (38.4%) | 689 (25.0%) |
| Yes | 1,321 (85.7%) | 750 (61.6%) | 2,071 (75.0%) |
| Social media | | | |
| No | 660 (42.8%) | 592 (48.6%) | 1,252 (45.4%) |
| Yes | 882 (57.2%) | 626 (51.4%) | 1,508 (54.6%) |
| Diversity of daily media consumption | | | |
| None | 46 (3.0%) | 63 (5.2%) | 109 (3.9%) |
| One-sided: Social media (Some) | 35 (2.3%) | 25 (2.1%) | 60 (2.2%) |
| One-sided: Broadcast | 60 (3.9%) | 183 (15.0%) | 243 (8.8%) |
| One-sided: Print | 75 (4.9%) | 32 (2.6%) | 107 (3.9%) |
| Two-sided | 657 (42.6%) | 548 (45.0%) | 1,205 (43.7%) |
| Three-sided | 669 (43.4%) | 367 (30.1%) | 1,036 (37.5%) |
| Gender | | | |
| Female | 798 (51.8%) | 561 (46.1%) | 1,359 (49.2%) |
| Male | 744 (48.2%) | 657 (53.9%) | 1,401 (50.8%) |
| Education | | | |
| Primary/secondary | 733 (48.1%) | 481 (39.5%) | 1,214 (44.3%) |
| Bachelor/college | 516 (33.9%) | 489 (40.1%) | 1,005 (36.7%) |
| Master | 274 (18.0%) | 248 (20.4%) | 522 (19.0%) |
| *N* | 1,542 (55.9%) | 1,218 (44.1%) | 2,760 (100.0%) |

## 74   Aki Koivula et al.

in combination, allowing us to differentiate between respondents who did not consume media daily, those who consumed only one media platform daily, and those who consumed two or three platforms daily.

Throughout the analysis, we considered the control variables sex, age, and education (see the Appendix).

### Analysis Procedure

We employed STATA version 17.0 for all statistical analyses and adopted a hierarchical data approach, recognizing that individuals were nested within both time points and countries. We conducted separate analyses for Finnish and US respondents and applied random-effect within–between models (REWB) to account for the correlated structure of panel data in our regression analyses. To achieve this, we utilized the *mixed* command with clustered standard errors to model both between-person and within-person effects over time while introducing control variables simultaneously. This process involved generating cluster-specific means and deviation scores of independent variables, which enabled us to obtain between- and within-individual effects, respectively. A key advantage of using REWB models was the ability to estimate between-subject effects simultaneously with level-one within-effect estimates, utilizing all cases (Bell et al., 2019). Additionally, we focused on individual media platforms by conducting an interaction analysis to isolate the significance of each platform and assess whether one-sided media consumption, particularly social media-focused, was associated with decreased trust in experts. We also examined differences in media effects between countries, conducting separate analyses for each.

### Results

Fig. 5.1 depicts the distribution of central variables in both countries at both measurement points. Notably, trust in experts was considerably higher in Finland than in the United States at the second measurement point. Of particular importance is the observation that in Finland, trust remained consistent across rounds, with roughly 75% expressing trust (at level 4 or 5) in experts' ability to solve the crisis at T1, while the proportion of confident respondents increased only slightly to 77.8% at T2. By contrast, in the United States, the corresponding proportions were 74.1% and 67.3% at T1 and T2, respectively, indicating differing trends in trust across the countries.

In the spring and autumn of 2020, Finns reported higher levels of satisfaction with government actions compared to their US counterparts. Specifically, 66.4% and 59.3% of Finns were satisfied with their government's actions in the spring and autumn of 2020, respectively, whereas only 43.2% and 32.5% of Americans reported satisfaction. Additionally, the degree of dissatisfaction with government actions increased more sharply in the United States than in Finland. Although media consumption patterns remained stable in both countries between spring and autumn, there was a significant discrepancy in print media consumption. Specifically, a higher proportion of Finns (87.3% and 84% in spring and autumn, respectively) reported reading print media daily compared to their US counterparts (65.4% and 57.8% in spring and autumn, respectively).

Media Consumption and Government Satisfaction    75

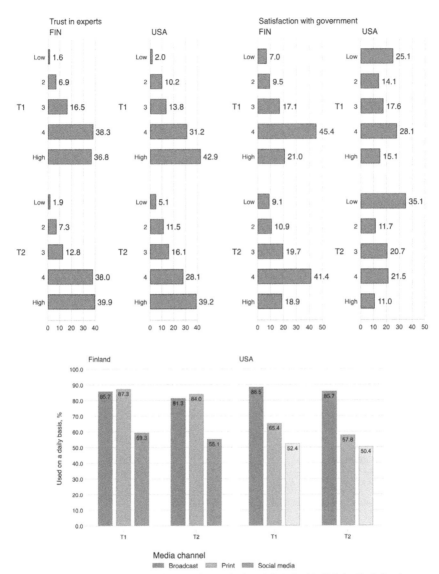

Fig. 5.1.   Trust in Experts' Capability to Solve COVID-19 Crisis, Satisfaction with Government Response to COVID-19 Crisis, and Daily Media Consumption Patterns in Finland and the United States in the T1 and T2 (Percentages).

Table 5.2 presents the results of a multilevel analysis that reveals the varying effects of media consumption and government satisfaction across countries. In Finland, we observed a strong association between average satisfaction with government actions and trust in experts to solve the crisis. However, within individuals, we did not find a statistically significant relationship between an increase in satisfaction and expert trust (at $p<0.05$ level). In contrast, in the

## 76 Aki Koivula et al.

Table 5.2. Trust in Experts According to Satisfaction with Government, Media Consumption Patterns, and Control Variables..

| | Finland | | United States | |
|---|---|---|---|---|
| *Within-subject* | | | | |
| Satisfaction with government | 0.05 | (0.05) | 0.07 | (0.05) |
| Broadcast | 0.10 | (0.20) | −0.05 | (0.32) |
| Print | 0.00 | (0.19) | 0.66** | (0.22) |
| Social media | −0.05 | (0.18) | 0.20 | (0.22) |
| *Between-subject* | | | | |
| Satisfaction with government | 0.38*** | (0.03) | −0.18*** | (0.03) |
| Broadcast | −0.16 | (0.18) | 0.78* | (0.31) |
| Print | 0.89*** | (0.19) | 0.83*** | (0.19) |
| Social media | 0.01 | (0.12) | 0.36* | (0.17) |
| Female | 0.28** | (0.11) | 0.04 | (0.15) |
| Age | 0.01** | (0.00) | 0.02*** | (0.01) |
| College degree | 0.78*** | (0.14) | 0.54** | (0.17) |
| Constant | 3.24*** | (0.39) | 5.10*** | (0.53) |
| *Random effect parameters* | | | | |
| Intercept (ID) | 1.14 | (0.06) | 1.42 | (0.07) |
| Residual | 1.27 | (0.04) | 1.62 | (0.06) |
| *ICC* | 0.44 | | 0.43 | |
| Observations | 1,523 | | 1,218 | |
| Number of groups | 767 | | 609 | |

*** $p<0.001$, ** $p<0.01$, * $p<0.05$.

Note: Robust standard errors in parentheses. REWB models.

United States, government satisfaction was found to be negatively related to expert confidence across respondents, with no association observed within individuals. Fig. 5.2 highlights this varying importance of government satisfaction across countries, illustrating how in Finland, government satisfaction is positively associated with expert confidence, while in the United States, the relationship is the opposite.

The findings indicate that in Finland, individuals who consume print media daily are on average more trusting of experts, when comparing individuals. However, we did not detect a temporal association at the individual level. In the United States, *on* the other hand, we found that an increase in print media consumption over time was directly linked to an increase in trust in experts within individuals. Additionally, in the United States, overall daily media consumption, including

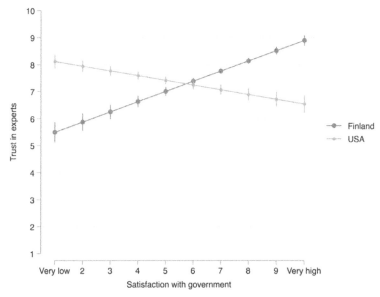

Fig. 5.2. Trust in Experts in Finland and the United States According to Satisfaction with Government Response to COVID-19 Crisis. *Note*: Predicted margins from the between-level effects estimated with the REWB models (Table 5.2).

print, social media, and broadcast media, was associated with increased trust in experts between individuals.

Additionally, we ran models in which the primary explanatory variables were independent of one another. Nevertheless, no statistically significant distinction was observed between these models and the overall effects we presented. Finally, we examined how the concentration and diversity of media consumption affect expert confidence. The results of the interaction analysis are presented in Fig. 5.3, which displays the mixed-effect results that consider both fixed and random effects simultaneously.

Our findings support our expectations that a greater emphasis on social media in daily consumption is associated with lower trust in experts in both countries. However, this association is considerably stronger in the United States than in Finland. Additionally, in the United States, a biased daily media consumption toward television also predicts lower trust, which cannot be observed in Finland.

## Discussion

This chapter focused on how media consumption patterns and government satisfaction predict views on scientific experts' capability to solve problems during a pandemic. The concept of trust has been a subject of considerable interest during the COVID-19 pandemic (Devine et al., 2024). However, previous studies have not focused on the construction of trust in experts. In this study, we examined

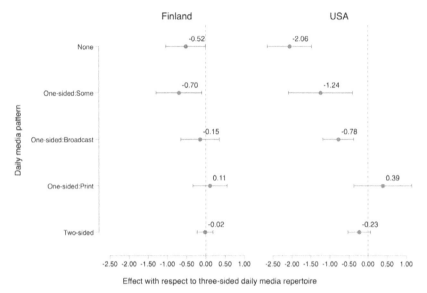

Fig. 5.3. The Effect of Daily Media Consumption Patterns on Trust in Experts. *Note*: The unstandardized coefficients with confidence intervals from the mixed linear regression models.

it from two different perspectives. First, we examined whether trust in experts is rooted to people's general views on the political context and governance during the crisis. Second, we considered the comprehensive nature of the media environment, which was much debated during the COVID-19 crisis. More specifically, our analytic strategy was to compare satisfaction with government and media consumption habits in the United States and Finland, and on this basis, estimate their impact on trust in experts.

The findings indicate a clear relationship between satisfaction with government actions and trust in experts during the crisis. However, it is notable that these relationships diverged significantly between Finland and the United States, underscoring the influence of both the political landscape and the cultural context during the crises. In Finland, satisfaction with the government was associated with increased trust in experts, whereas in the United States, the relationship was inverse: greater satisfaction with the government corresponded to diminished trust in experts. However, it is notable that we could not find the significant within-level effects in either country, which indicates that during this 6-month follow-up period, within-persons changes in satisfaction with the government were not found to be positively or negatively reflected in trust in experts' abilities.

The results also revealed divergent trends in media consumption patterns and trust in experts between Finland and the United States. While traditional journalistic print media consumption was associated with higher trust in experts in both countries, the results showed greater variability in trust levels in the United States based on daily media consumption across platforms. Additionally, the

## Media Consumption and Government Satisfaction  79

findings highlighted the potential negative impact of one-sided reliance on social media content, particularly evident in the United States, suggesting a need for a deeper understanding of the role of social media in shaping and maintaining trust dynamics.

One possible mechanism that could explain the differences in the outcomes of media usage patterns is the fact that users are exposed to different kinds of content in different media platforms. Traditional news media platforms, such as print media and television, have long traditions in presenting their content within certain formats, and journalistic practices regulate the information delivered by such platforms. For example, when journalists in newspaper share information about a specific event or an issue, they often employ well-established frames to offer interpretations about the issue at hand (e.g., de Vreese, 2005). Additionally, journalistic practices also affect the choices and adaptations regarding expertise: journalists select the experts to be interviewed, reformulate the content produced by the experts, and exclude some experts (Albæk, 2011). This variation in how the scientific information is presented and delivered is further complicated by the current media environment (Chadwick, 2017), where individuals are exposed to various, and often contradictory, explanations of the issue using different media channels.

During the pandemic, there were also concerns that spread of misleading information may delay authorities' and experts' efforts to deal with the crisis. Already before the pandemic, the spread of misinformation was recognized as a serious issue that can affect trust in experts. However, the politicization of the pandemic-related health information and other issues threatened citizens' trust in experts at several stages of the pandemic. This was seen especially in the United States, where experts had difficulties in correcting strongly politicized, wrongful information. Alternatively, Finland presents an opposite context in which public satisfaction with government is closely linked with trust in experts. This dynamic potentially improved the effectiveness of evidence-based policies during the pandemic.

In conclusion, this study underscores the critical role of diverse news sources and effective information dissemination during emergencies. It highlights the importance of using different media channels to build trust in expert institutions, and particularly emphasizes its relevance in the context of the United States compared to Finland. However, it is also important to recognize that trust in experts is closely linked with the dynamics of political governance and citizens' responses to it. Furthermore, the study acknowledges the existence of different content and knowledge on different platforms, a factor not fully explored here. Future research should explore platform-specific political polarization and its impact on trust to gain a more comprehensive understanding of media influence in emergency situations.

## References

Ahluwalia, S. C., Edelen, M. O., Qureshi, N., & Etchegaray, J. M. (2021). Trust in experts, not trust in national leadership, leads to greater uptake of recommended actions during the COVID-19 pandemic. *Risk, Hazards & Crisis in Public Policy, 12*(3), 283–302.

## 80 Aki Koivula et al.

Albæk, E. (2011). The interaction between experts and journalists in news journalism. *Journalism, 12*(3), 335–348. https://doi.org/10.1177/1464884910392851

Anderson, A. A., Scheufele, D. A., Brossard, D., & Corley, E. A. (2012). The role of media and deference to scientific authority in cultivating trust in sources of information about emerging technologies. *International Journal of Public Opinion Research, 24*(2), 225–237.

Avery, J. M. (2009). Videomalaise or virtuous circle? The influence of the news media on political trust. *The International Journal of Press/Politics, 14*(4), 410–433.

Baker, W. D., & Oneal, J. R. (2001). Patriotism or opinion leadership? The nature and origins of the "rally 'round the flag" effect. *Journal of Conflict Resolution, 45*(5), 661–687.

Balliet, D., & Van Lange, P. A. (2013). Trust, conflict, and cooperation: a meta-analysis. *Psychological Bulletin, 139*(5), 1090.

Ban, P., Park, J. Y., & You, H. Y. (2022). How are politicians informed? Witnesses and information provision in congress. *American Political Science Review, 117*(1), 122–139.

Bargain, O., & Aminjonov, U. (2020). Trust and compliance to public health policies in times of COVID-19. *Journal of Public Economics, 192*(1), 104316.

Baum, M. A. (2002). The constituent foundations of the rally-round-the-flag phenomenon. International Studies Quarterly, *46*(2), 263–298.

Bell, A., Fairbrother, M., & Jones, K. (2019). Fixed and random effects models: Making an informed choice. *Quality & Quantity, 54*(1), 1051–1074.

Bollyky, T. J., Hulland, E. N., Barber, R. M., Collins, J. K., Kiernan, S., Moses, M., Pigott, D. M., Reiner, R. C, Sorensen, R. J. D, Abbafati, C., Adolph, C, Allorant, J. O. A., Aravkin, A. Y., Bang-Jensen, B., Carter, A., Castellano, R., Castro, E., Chakrabarti, S., Combs, E., & Dieleman, J. L. (2022). Pandemic preparedness and COVID-19: an exploratory analysis of infection and fatality rates, and contextual factors associated with preparedness in 177 countries, from Jan 1, 2020, to Sept 30, 2021. *The Lancet, 399*(10334), 1489–1512.

Brader, T., Tucker, J. A., & Duell, D. (2013). Which parties can lead opinion? Experimental evidence on partisan cue taking in multiparty democracies. *Comparative Political Studies, 46*(11), 1485–1517.

Braithwaite, J., & Makkai, T. (1994), Trust and compliance. *Policing and Society: An International Journal, 4*(1), 1–12.

Cairney, P., & Wellstead, A. (2021). COVID-19: effective policymaking depends on trust in experts, politicians, and the public. *Policy Design and Practice, 4*(1), 1–14.

Chadwick, A. (2017). *The hybrid media system: Politics and power*. Oxford University Press.

Chan, A. K., Nickson, C. P., Rudolph, J. W., Lee, A., & Joynt, G. M. (2020). Social media for rapid knowledge dissemination: Early experience from the COVID-19 pandemic. *Anaesthesia, 75*(12), 1579.

Cheung, C. K., & Tse, J. W. L. (2008). Institutional trust as a determinant of anxiety during the SARS crisis in Hong Kong. *Social Work in Public Health, 23*(5), 41–54.

Citrin, J., & Stoker, L. (2018). Political trust in a cynical age. *Annual Review of Political Science, 21*(1), 49–70.

Coleman, J. S. (1988). Social capital in the creation of human capital. *American Journal of Sociology, 94*, 95–120.

Cuello-Garcia, C., Pérez-Gaxiola, G., & van Amelsvoort, L. (2020). Social media can have an impact on how we manage and investigate the COVID-19 pandemic. *Journal of Clinical Epidemiology, 127*, 198–201.

Devine, D., Valgarðsson, V., Smith, J., Jennings, W., Scotto di Vettimo, M., Bunting, H., & McKay, L. (2024). Political trust in the first year of the COVID-19 pandemic: A meta-analysis of 67 studies. *Journal of European Public Policy, 31*(3), 657–679.

de Vreese, C. H. (2005). News framing: Theory and typology. *Information Desing Journal + Document Design, 13*(1), 51–62.

## Media Consumption and Government Satisfaction    81

Druckman, J. N., Peterson, E., & Slothuus, R. (2013). How elite partisan polarization affects public opinion formation. *American Political Science Review, 107*(1), 57–79.

Dudo, A., Brossard, D., Shanahan, J., Scheufele, D. A., Morgan, M., & Signorielli, N. (2011). Science on television in the 21st century: Recent trends in portrayals and their contributions to public attitudes toward science. *Communication Research, 38*(6), 754–777.

Granovetter, M. (1985). Economic action and social structure: The problem of embeddedness. *American Journal of Sociology, 91*(3), 481–510.

Gross, K., Aday, S., & Brewer, P. R. (2004). A panel study of media effects on political and social trust after September 11, 2001. *Harvard International Journal of Press/Politics, 9*(4), 49–73.

Hetherington, M. J. (1998). The political relevance of political trust. *American Political Science Review, 92*(4), 791–808.

Hetherington, M. J., & Nelson, M. (2003). Anatomy of a rally effect: George W. Bush and the war on terrorism. *PS: Political Science & Politics, 36*(1), 37–42.

Hmielowski, J. D., Feldman, L., Myers, T. A., Leiserowitz, A., & Maibach, E. (2014). An attack on science? Media use, trust in scientists, and perceptions of global warming. *Public Understanding of Science, 23*(7), 866–883. https://doi.org/10.1177/0963662513480091

Huber, B., Barnidge, M., Gil de Zúñiga, H., & Liu, J. (2019). Fostering public trust in science: The role of social media. *Public Understanding of Science, 28*(7), 759–777.

Jarreau, P. B., Cancellare, I. A., Carmichael, B. J., Porter, L., Toker, D., & Yammine, S. Z. (2019). Using selfies to challenge public stereotypes of scientists. *PloS One, 14*(5), e0216625.

Kestilä-Kekkonen, E., Koivula, A., & Tiihonen, A. (2022). When trust is not enough. A longitudinal analysis of political trust and political competence during the first wave of the COVID-19 pandemic in Finland. *European Political Science Review, 14*(3), 424–440.

Klein, E., & Robinson, J. (2020). Like, post, and distrust? How social media use affects trust in government. *Political Communication, 37*(1), 46–64. https://doi.org/10.1080/10584609.2019.1661891

Laor, T., & Lissitsa, S. (2022). Mainstream, on-demand and social media consumption and trust in government handling of the COVID crisis. *Online Information Review, 46*(7), 1335–1352. https://doi.org/10.1108/OIR

Levi, M., & Stoker, L. (2000). Political trust and trustworthiness. *Annual Review of Political Science, 3*(1), 475–507.

Luhmann, N. (1979). Trust and power. John Wiley & Sons.

Macy, M. W., & Skvoretz, J. (1998). The evolution of trust and cooperation between strangers: A computational model. *American Sociological Review, 63*(5), 638–660.

Majid, U., Wasim, A., Truong, J., & Bakshi, S. (2021). Public trust in governments, health care providers, and the media during pandemics: A systematic review. *Journal of Trust Research, 11*(2), 119–141.

Mayer, J. D. (2020). The contemporary presidency: Two presidents, two crises: Bush Wrestles with 9/11, Trump Fumbles COVID-19. *Presidential Studies Quarterly, 50*(3), 629–649.

Mayer, R. C., Davis, J. H., & Schoorman, F. D. (1995). An integrative model of organizational trust. *Academy of Management Review, 20*(3), 709–734.

McFall, L. (1987). Integrity. *Ethics, 98*(1), 5–20.

Mihelj, S., Kondor, K., & Štětka, V. (2022). Establishing trust in experts during a crisis: Expert trustworthiness and media use during the COVID-19 pandemic. *Science Communication, 44*(3), 292–319.

Miller, C. (2001). Hybrid management: Boundary organizations, science policy, and environmental governance in the climate regime. *Science, Technology, & Human Values, 26*(4), 478–500.

## 82 Aki Koivula et al.

Mueller, J. E. (1970). Presidential Popularity from Truman to Johnson. *American Political Science Review, 64*(1), 18–34.

Nisbet, M. C., Scheufele, D. A., Shanahan, J., Moy, P., Brossard, D., & Lewenstein, B. V. (2002). Knowledge, reservations, or promise? A media effects model for public perceptions of science and technology. *Communication Research, 29*(5), 584–609. https://doi.org/10.1177/009365002236196

Oksanen, A., Kaakinen, M., Latikka, R., Savolainen, I., Savela, N., & Koivula, A. (2020). Regulation and trust: 3-month follow-up study on COVID-19 mortality in 25 European countries. *JMIR Public Health and Surveillance, 6*(2), e19218.

Olsson, E. K., & Nord, L. W. (2015). Paving the way for crisis exploitation: The role of journalistic styles and standards. *Journalism, 16*(3), 341–358. https://doi.org/ 10.1177/1464884913519032

Pechar, E., Bernauer, T., & Mayer, F. (2018). Beyond political ideology: The impact of attitudes towards government and corporations on trust in science. *Science Communication, 40*(3), 291–313.

Pink, S. L., Chu, J., Druckman, J. N., Rand, D. G., & Willer, R. (2021). Elite party cues increase vaccination intentions among Republicans. *Proceedings of the National Academy of Sciences, 118*(2), e2106559118.

Plohl, N., & Musil, B. (2021). Modeling compliance with COVID-19 prevention guidelines: The critical role of trust in science. *Psychology, Health & Medicine, 26*(1), 1–12.

PytlikZillig, L. M., & Kimbrough, C. D. (2016). Consensus on conceptualizations and definitions of trust: Are we there yet?. In E. Shockley, T. M. Neal, L. M. PytlikZillig, & B. H. Bornstein (Eds.), *Interdisciplinary perspectives on trust* (pp. 17–47). Springer.

Reif, A., Kneisel, T., Schäfer, M., & Taddicken, M. (2020). Why are scientific experts perceived as trustworthy? Emotional assessment within TV and YouTube videos. *Media and Communication, 8*(1), 191–205.

Robbins, B. G. (2016). What is trust? A multidisciplinary review, critique, and synthesis. *Sociology Compass, 10*(10), 972–986.

Rousseau, D. M., Sitkin, S. B., Burt, R. S., & Camerer, C. (1998). Not so different after all: A cross-discipline view of trust. *Academy of Management Review, 23*(3), 393–404.

Saarinen, A., Koivula, A., & Keipi, T. (2020). Political trust, political party preference and trust in knowledge-based institutions. *International Journal of Sociology and Social Policy, 40*(1/2), 154–168.

Schilke, O., Reimann, M., & Cook, K. S. (2021). Trust in social relations. *Annual Review of Sociology, 47*(1), 239–259.

Sitkin, S. B., & Roth, N. L. (1993). Explaining the limited effectiveness of legalistic remedies for trust/distrust. *Organization Science, 4*(3), 367–392.

Slothuus, R. (2016). Assessing the influence of political parties on public opinion: The challenge from pretreatment effects. *Political Communication, 33*(2), 302–327.

Slovic, P., & Weber, E. U. (2002, April 12–13). *Perception of risk posed by extreme events* [Paper presentation]. Risk management strategies in an uncertain world conference, Palisades, New York.

Strömbäck, J., Djerf-Pierre, M., & Shehata, A. (2016). A question of time? A longitudinal analysis of the relationship between news media consumption and political trust. *International Journal of Press/Politics, 21*(1), 88–110. https://doi.org/ 10.1177/1940161215613059

Sztompka, P. (1999). *Trust: A sociological theory*. Cambridge University Press.

Van der Meer, T., & Hakhverdian, A. (2017). Political trust as the evaluation of process and performance: A cross-national study of 42 European countries. *Political Studies, 65*(1), 81–102.

Van Dijck, J., & Alinejad, D. (2020). Social media and trust in scientific expertise: Debating the Covid-19 pandemic in the Netherlands. *Social Media+ Society*, 6(4), 2056305120981057.

Vos, J. (2021). *The psychology of COVID-19: Building resilience for future pandemics* (1st ed.). SAGE.

Wynen, J., Op de Beeck, S., Verhoest, K., Glavina, M., Six, F., Van Damme, P., Beutels, P., Hedrickx, G., & Pepermans, K. (2022). Taking a COVID-19 vaccine or not? Do trust in government and trust in experts help us to understand vaccination intention?. *Administration & Society*, 54(10), 1875–1901.

Zarolia, P., Weisbuch, M., & McRae, K. (2017). Influence of indirect information on interpersonal trust despite direct information. *Journal of Personality and Social Psychology*, 112(1), 39–57.

Chapter 6

# COVID-19 and the Flames of Hate

*James Hawdon*

*Virginia Tech, USA*

## Abstract

This chapter examines how the pandemic altered exposure to online hate. We investigate if the pandemic affected previously observed patterns of exposure to online hate in Finland and the United States. We ask, did online hate become more prevalent as the pandemic unfolded and became increasingly politicized? It is important to consider online hate exposure in the early stages of the pandemic because the pandemic fanned the flames of hate. This increase in hate can then lead to fewer people complying with recommended health-protective behaviors and increases in hate crimes, which would increase the overall toll of the pandemic. Thus, this chapter explores if the landscape of online hate in the United States and Finland changed in the initial stages of COVID-19. Initially, rates of exposure were higher in Finland than in the United States, and, as predicted, rates of exposure increased between April and November 2020. However, this increase was observed only in the United States. The increase in exposure in the United States combined with the stability in exposure in Finland resulted in the country differences that were observed in April disappearing by November. The chapter concludes by exploring the likely role of the political leaders of the two nations played in this pattern of online hate exposure. Specifically, President Trump's use of racialized descriptions of the pandemic are contrast to Prime Minister Marion's more scientific descriptions to demonstrate how policy rhetoric can encourage or discourage online hate.

*Keywords*: Online hate; hate crime; anti-Asian hate; COVID-19 and hate; cross-national comparisons of hate

---

Perceptions of a Pandemic: A Cross-Continental Comparison of Citizen Perceptions,
Attitudes, and Behaviors During COVID-19, 85–104
Copyright © 2025 by James Hawdon
Published under exclusive licence by Emerald Publishing Limited
doi:10.1108/978-1-83608-624-620241006

## 86  James Hawdon

## Introduction

The COVID-19 pandemic upended society in ways that have not been experienced for generations. While other recent pandemics had devastating effects, they did not shut down the global economy. While pandemics vary in terms of geographic scope, degrees of contagion, methods of contagion, and deadliness, one thing most pandemics have in common is that they stoke fear. Fear is common and especially pronounced in the earliest stages of the pandemic when it is often the case that little is known about the nature of the disease, how it is transmitted, and how we can protect ourselves against it. The COVID-19 pandemic resembled many other pandemics in this way as it undoubtedly triggered fear throughout the population. As the disease's seriousness became all too evident, people became increasingly fearful for their lives and the lives of their loved ones. As noted in Chapter 2, 94.2% of Americans and 92.2% of Finns said they were at least slightly concerned about the pandemic.

Fear, of course, is a normal and extremely useful emotion. Indeed, it is programmed into our nervous system and results from biochemical reactions, which produces an automatic "fight or flight" response to real or perceived threats. Fear alerts us to dangers, heightens our awareness, sharpens our focus, and makes us take precautions. It is critical for our survival and in many situations can save our lives. Yet too much fear is obviously detrimental to our well-being. It can paralyze us at times, and it can be a symptom of serious mental health conditions including panic disorder, phobias, or post-traumatic stress disorder. Too much fear and the stress that results from it can also lead to serious health problems. Fear can also have profound consequences at the community level. As is well documented, widespread fear can create an atmosphere conducive to hate. Indeed, even at the interpersonal level, hate is a secondary emotion that arises from fear, including the fear of mortality (Shapiro, 2016), and fear is central to numerous theories of hate (e.g., Lake & Rothchild, 1998; McCaulley, 2016; Sternberg, 2020; Suny, 2004).

Given the fear induced by COVID-19, it is reasonable to suspect that hate increased during the pandemic. In this chapter, we explore if there is evidence that occurred. We begin by reviewing the nature of hate in the United States and Finland using available data. We consider survey data from previously published works from other scholars as was as data from this project to see if respondents reported seeing hateful content while online and if the extent to which they were exposed to such content increased during our study period. We then consider the cross-national differences and possible reasons that can explain the differences we observe. These differences will highlight why it is critical to understand the role that exposure to hate can play during a pandemic.

## The Importance of Online Hate

Online hate expresses hatred of some collective (see Blazak, 2009; Hawdon et al., 2014, 2017) by devaluing the group because of their religion, race, ethnicity, gender, sexual orientation, national origin, or some other characteristic that defines the group. The collective focus of online hate distinguishes it from individualized

COVID-19 and the Flames of Hate     **87**

forms of cyberviolence, such as cyberstalking or cyberbullying (Costello et al., 2016). Although online hate materials can target specific individuals, such materials would be considered online hate only if the targeted individuals were systemically devaluated by virtue of being a member of a collective. Online hate can range from stereotyping, to attributing personal or societal problems to a group, to advocating discrimination or violence against a group (Hawdon et al., 2019; Phadke et al., 2018).

Organized hate groups such as the Klu Klux Klan established an online presence almost immediately after the Internet's invention (Bowman-Grieve, 2009), and the number of sites and methods for advocating hate has increased considerably over time. With the advent of social networking platforms such as Facebook and Twitter, it became extremely easy to create and disseminate hate materials (Potok, 2015). Moreover, the days of hate materials being hosted on static webpages have passed and more interactive forums that allow materials to be shaped through communal debate now dominate virtual spaces (Snow et al., 2013). As with terrorism, online hate is created and disseminated by those on both the political right and political left, and it can focus on a single group (e.g., Muslims, Mexicans, women), a single issue (e.g., immigration, gay rights, environmental policy), or a more general issue such as the pandemic (see Southern Poverty Law Center, 2017). Currently, a disproportionate amount of online hate expresses rightwing views, and rightwing extremists who promulgate racist, misogynistic, hyper-nationalistic, anti-government, and/or anti-immigrant ideas are the most active producers of online hate (Costello & Hawdon, 2020; Hawdon et al., 2019; Southern Poverty Law Center, 2017). This is true in both Finland and the United States, and it is true in other European nations as well (Reichelmann et al., 2021).

While online hate can be vile and disturbing, we must be careful not to overstate the adverse effects of seeing online hate. In fact, the effect that exposure to online hate has on an individual is unquestionably dependent on factors such as whether the exposure is deliberate or not and if the exposed person agrees with the ideologies professed in the materials. As noted by Costello and Hawdon (2020), exposure to hate materials is not necessarily *victimizing*, at least in the traditional sense. Those who actively search for these materials and those who agree with them would not be "victims" in the traditional sense of the term. Still others who see these materials do not experience negative consequences, even if they disagree with them or find them extremely offensive (Costello & Hawdon, 2020). Thus, online hate does not necessarily harm everyone who sees it.

Nevertheless, while recognizing that not everyone who is exposed to these materials is victimized by them in the traditional sense, there is growing evidence that online hate is problematic (e.g., Keipi et al., 2017). For example, exposure to hate materials can decrease the viewer's sense of general well-being (Keipi et al., 2017). Exposure to hate can also reinforce discriminatory attitudes against targeted groups (Foxman & Wolf, 2013; Soral et al., 2018) while simultaneously increasing fear among members of targeted groups (Tynes, 2006). Exposure to online hate can also undermine social trust (Näsi et al., 2015) and faith in social institutions (Hawdon et al., 2019). Online hate has also been linked to radicalization (Holt et al., 2019), and in extreme cases, exposure can lead to acts of offline

## 88 James Hawdon

violence (see Costello & Hawdon, 2020; Federal Bureau of Investigation (FBI), 2011; Freilich et al., 2011; Lu & Sheng, 2020; The New America Foundation International Security Program, 2015). These last effects concern us most when it comes to online hate and the COVID-19 pandemic.

## The Importance of Online Hate During the COVID-19 Pandemic

First, as noted above, rightwing hate is by far the most prominent form of online hate today, and, given the prevalence of this type of hate, the likelihood of viewing it is relatively high. Much of this hate advocates a deep mistrust of government and other social institutions, and much of it is designed to promote conspiracy theories (Southern Poverty Law Center, 2022). Because social media creates "filter bubbles" whereby users' preferences are parroted back to them and they are increasingly funneled into groups of like-minded people (Pariser, 2011), those whose views even remotely align with political messages being offered will increasingly see additional content expressing similar or increasingly extreme attitudes. This process narrows and polarizes the messages being seen (Hawdon, 2012; also see Keipi et al., 2017; Pariser, 2011), and this further increases the likelihood of seeing these messages again (Hawdon et al., 2019). The more people see these ideas expressed and collectively approved by those in their narrowing filter bubble, the greater the likelihood that such extremist positions begin to appear legitimate and to be widely held. This is relevant for the pandemic because, as seen in previous research (Bish & Michie, 2010; Choi & Fox, 2022; Doogan et al., 2020; Kestilä-Kekkonen et al., 2022; Sedgwick et al., 2022) and discussed in later chapters, trust and confidence in the government increase compliance with governmentally suggested health-protective behaviors. Given that complying with these recommendations saved lives (e.g., Howard et al., 2021; Miyazawa & Kaneko, 2020; Motallebi et al., 2022), widespread exposure to hate can indirectly increase the severity of COVID-19 by decreasing compliance with health-protective behaviors.

Next, exposure to online hate is also relevant because it is associated with increases in offline violence. There is growing evidence that online materials can radicalize individuals and, in extreme cases, lead to violence. While this pathway to violence remains fortunately rare, it is seemingly increasing as a growing number of horrific acts of mass violence have been linked to online radicalization (see Costello & Hawdon, 2020; Lu & Sheng, 2020). Indeed, although data on hate crimes are woefully insufficient and official statistics undoubtedly underestimate the amount of hate crime that occurs, it is clear that such acts have recently increased throughout much of Europe and the United States during the pandemic.[1] For example, in the United States, reported hate crimes increased

---

[1]Hate crimes are defined by the FBI as criminal offense against a person or property motivated in whole or in part by an offender's bias against a race, religion, disability, sexual orientation, ethnicity, gender, or gender identity (FBI, 2011).

COVID-19 and the Flames of Hate    *89*

from 7,314 reported incidents in 2019 to 8,263 in 2020 to 10,840 in 2021, an increase of 48.2%. This increase in reported incidents was recorded despite 452 fewer agencies reporting to the FBI (US Department of Justice, 2020, 2021). A similar increase was witnessed in Finland. The number of reported hate crimes increased by approximately 30% in 2020 compared to 2019, increasing from 900 to 1,177. The number of reported hate crimes reported to Finnish authorities increased again in 2021 by an additional 18%, rising to 1,390 incidents. Therefore, over the course of the pandemic's first two years, Finland witnessed a 54.4% increase in hate crimes recorded by police. In both the United States and Finland – and indeed in most nations that report to ODIHR – most hate crimes are rooted in racism and xenophobia (OSCE, 2022), which is also the most common form of online hate in both countries (Reichelmann et al., 2021).

Again, not everyone – or even most – who sees online hate will go on to commit a hate crime; however, there is evidence that increases in exposure to online hate correspond to increases in offline hate crimes (Hawdon et al., 2022). For example, Chan et al. (2016) found that broadband availability increases racial hate crimes in areas with a high proportion of racially derogatory Google search terms. Similarly, anti-refugee sentiments on Facebook predict anti-refugee hate crimes (Müller & Schwarz, 2021). Thus, while the likelihood of someone viewing online hate committing a hate crime may be low, there is a connection between visceral online hate and performing acts of violence offline.

Therefore, it is important to look at online hate exposure in the initial stages of the pandemic because it may have fanned the flames of hate and led to more online hate being viewed. This increase in hate, in turn, can then lead to fewer people complying with recommended health-protective behaviors and increases in hate crimes. Both outcomes would increase the overall toll the pandemic had on the American and Finnish societies. We therefore ask, "What was the landscape of online hate in the United States and Finland before the pandemic and how did this landscape change in the early stages of COVID-19?"

## Landscape of Online Hate in Finland and the United States

Previous research indicates that both Finland and the United States have comparatively high levels of exposure to hate. In 2013, when a sample of youth and young adults ages 15–30 from Finland, Germany, the United States, and the United Kingdom were asked if they had seen hateful materials online that attacked certain groups of people or individuals, Finland and the United States had significantly higher rates of exposure than did the other two nations. Approximately 55% of American and 48% of Finnish respondents reported seeing such materials. By comparison, only 38% of respondents from the United Kingdom and 31% of German respondents reported seeing such materials (see Hawdon et al., 2015, 2017). These differences remained even after controlling for individual-level factors known to be related to exposure. When looking at the percentage of respondents who reported being targeted by such messages, over 16% of American youth and young people reported being targets of online hate. Youth from the United Kingdom (12%) and Finland (10%) reported significantly lower rates of

## 90 *James Hawdon*

targeting, and only 4% of German respondents reported being targets of online hate (Hawdon et al., 2015).

Using 2018 data from young adults 18–25, Reichelmann et al. (2021) also found that online hate exposure was comparatively high in the United States and Finland. In this sample, Finland had the highest rates of exposure as over 78% of Finns reported seeing hateful or degrading writings or speech within three months of being surveyed. The next highest rates were reported for Spain (75%), the United States (73%), and Poland (72%). Respondents from the United Kingdom (66%) and France (65%) also reported relatively high rates of exposure to online hate; however, these rates were significantly lower than were those reported in the other nations. Moreover, when asked the frequency with which they see online hate materials, nearly 24% of respondents from the United States and 20% of those from Finland said they saw such materials frequently. By comparison, only 15% of Spanish respondents and approximately 10% of Polish respondents said they saw online hate material frequently (Reichelmann et al., 2021). Thus, most American and Finnish youth see online hate, and these youth are more likely than youth from many other European nations to see such materials frequently. Again, these national differences hold even after controlling for common individual-level factors that are correlated with online hate exposure (Reichelmann et al., 2021).

One plausible reason that the United States has comparatively high levels of exposure to online hate material is its relatively lax hate speech laws. While all the nations discussed above have legal provisions that protect free speech, the Constitution of the United States places legal primacy on protecting speech. Although speech can be limited for reasons of defamation, obscenity, and certain forms of state censorship, the courts have not made an exception for hate speech (see Bleich, 2011). Given the legal standards required to limit speech, the First Amendment and recent interpretations of it effectively eliminate hate speech regulation in the United States (Allen & Norris, 2011; Bleich, 2011). It is therefore unsurprising that Americans are exposed to a lot of online hate material. By comparison, Finland does have regulations banning hate speech. For example, Finland's Criminal Code (Ministry of Justice Finland, 2012: Section 10: 511/2011) outlaws the expressing of opinions "where a certain group is threatened, defamed or insulted on the basis of its race, skin color, birth status, national or ethnic origin, religion or belief, sexual orientation or disability or a comparable basis," as well as "aggravated ethnic agitation." While these laws are similar to those found in the United Kingdom and other European nations, these laws are infrequently enforced in Finland. For example, between 2000 and 2013, only 25 cases of ethnic agitation were reported, and those convicted only faced minor fines (see Hawdon et al., 2017, for details). Consequently, both the United States and Finland have a legal landscape that either explicitly allows or practically tolerates hate speech, including online hate.

Even though online hate has flourished in both the United States and Finland for well over a decade prior to the pandemic, we ask if the pandemic affected the rates of exposure to online hate. There are several reasons to suspect that exposure to online hate would increase during the early stages of the pandemic. First, as noted above, the pandemic was scary and created an atmosphere of fear, and

COVID-19 and the Flames of Hate    91

fear, in turn, often leads to hate. This phenomenon could particularly play out with a viral pandemic caused by person-to-person contact. As concern for our lives and the lives of others increase, the fear of others who may cause deadly harm can easily lead to the hatred of those others. If this hatred is generalized from individuals to groups of individuals – such as immigrants, specific ethnic groups, or particular sexual orientations – hatred of that group will increase, and online expressions of that hate will undoubtedly follow.

A second reason that exposure to hate would be expected to increase during the pandemic is peoples' online activities influence the likelihood they will be exposed to hate (e.g., Costello et al., 2016, 2019, 2020, 2021; Keipi et al., 2017). According to routine activity theory (Cohen & Felson, 1979), crime occurs with the convergence of a motivated offender, a suitable target, and a lack of capable guardianship that could prevent the crime from occurring. Applying this insight to online hate exposure, research reveals that those who spend more time online (Costello et al., 2020; Keipi et al., 2017), frequently visit social networking sites (Costello et al., 2021), regularly express opinions online (Hawdon et al., 2019), join in online attacks against others, and routinely discuss private matters online (Costello et al., 2021) are more likely to be exposed to online hate than are their counterparts. Given that the pandemic radically disrupted our daily lives and forced more people to spend more time online, our cyber-routines changed, and we would anticipate these changes would increase rates of exposure to online hate.[2]

## Online Hate During the COVID-19 Pandemic in Finland and the United States

To determine exposure to online hate materials, we asked respondents if they had seen "hateful or degrading writing or speech online inappropriately attacking individuals or groups" during the 3 months prior to being surveyed. We used this measure because it is the same question used to measure online hate exposure in numerous studies of online hate (e.g., Hawdon et al., 2014; Keipi et al., 2017), and we wanted our results to be as comparable as possible to this earlier work. Although we cannot make exact comparisons because many previous studies included minors and ours do not, we nevertheless believe the comparisons we can make are informative.

In the pandemic's early stages, a substantial percentage of respondents in both nations reported seeing online hate in the 3 months prior to the survey. In April 2020 when the first wave of data was collected, 1,180 (39.3%) of respondents reported seeing online hate materials. Like other multi-national studies (Reichelmann et al., 2021), Finnish respondents were more likely to report seeing online hate material than were American respondents. Whereas 647 of 1,500 Finnish respondents reported seeing hate materials, only 533 of 1,500 American respondents reported seeing hate (43.1% and 35.5%, respectively), which is a

---

[2]For a discussion of how online routine activities were changed by the pandemic, see Hawdon et al. (2020) and Gartner (2020).

statistically significant difference.[3] These rates are reported in Fig. 6.1. As noted above, Reichelmann and colleagues also reported Finnish respondents having higher levels of exposure than did Americans.[4]

To place these rates of exposure into perspective, the overall levels reported in our sample are similar to those reported by Hawdon et al. (2017). In that work, which used the same measure of exposure, Americans were more exposed than were Finns. Moreover, they reported higher overall rates of exposure (their 53% of Americans compared to our 35% and their 48% of Finns compared to our 43%). However, when we limit our sample to those under 30 to better match the sample they used, we get remarkably similar levels of exposure, albeit with the countries reversing their relative positions. Among our respondents who were 30 or younger, 55.8% (168 of 301) of Finns and 46.0% (157 of 341) of Americans reported seeing hate at the beginning of the pandemic. Although the earlier sample is not directly comparable because it also included youth ages 15–17, these numbers suggest that rates of exposure were not particularly elevated at the onset of the pandemic.

Fig. 6.2 reports rates of exposure in each country for those 30 and under in our sample, and those reported from an earlier study (e.g., Hawdon et al., 2017). As can be seen in the figure, Finland and the United States switched positions in

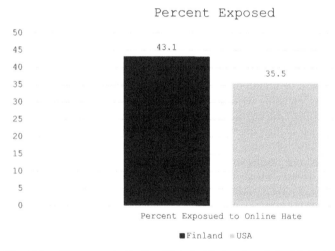

Fig. 6.1. Exposure to Online Hate in Finland and the United States: 2020.

---

[3]The difference between the countries was statistically significant ($\chi^2 = 18.15$; $p < 0.001$).

[4]Reichelmann and colleagues report much higher levels of exposure, with 78% of Finns and 73% of Americans reporting seeing hateful materials; however, those researchers used a different measure of hate. They asked, "In the past three months, have you seen hateful or degrading writings or speech online that attacked certain groups of people or individuals" (Reichelmann et al., 2021, p. 1102).

COVID-19 and the Flames of Hate 93

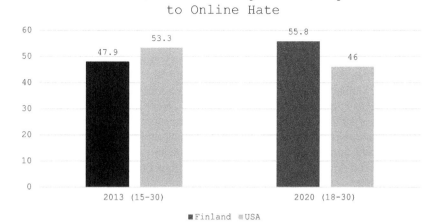

Fig. 6.2. Exposure to Online Hate in Finland and the United States Among Young: 2013 and 2020.

terms of which nation had the highest rate of exposure, but overall, approximately half of people under 30 in these two nations saw hate in 2013 and approximately half of similar aged respondents reported seeing it at the beginning of the pandemic.

Assuming rates of exposure were relatively unaffected at the earliest stages of the pandemic, we investigate if these rates changed as the pandemic unfolded. As predicted, rates of exposure did increase by November 2020 as compared to April 2020. By November, 42.8% of the total sample (1,329 of 3,035) reported seeing online hate materials compared to the 39% reporting this in April. This represents a statistically significant increase of 8.9% in exposure in a little over seven months.[5] However, this increase was observed only in the United States. In the United States, rates of exposure significantly increased from 35.5% of respondents to 41.4% of respondents between April and November. By comparison, rates of exposure barely changed between April and November in Finland, going from 43.1% in April to 44.1% in November.[6] The increase in exposure in the United States combined with the stability in exposure in Finland resulted in the country differences that were observed in April disappearing by November. That is, by the time our data were collected in November, the two nations had similar rates of exposure. Whereas 41.4% of Americans were exposed in November, 44.1%

---

[5]This increase was statistically significant ($\chi^2 = 7.41; p = 0.006$).
[6]The increase in exposure in the United States between April and November 2020 was statistically significant ($\chi^2 = 10.91; p < 0.001$). The change in Finland between April and November was not significant ($\chi^2 = 0.30; p = 0.582$).

## 94   James Hawdon

of Finns were, which is not a statistically significant difference.[7] Fig. 6.3 reports these results graphically.

Interestingly, the greater exposure to online hate observed in the American sample was driven by those over the age of 25. When the analysis is limited to young people between the ages of 18 and 25, there was no difference in exposure between April and November in either country. Among young Finns, 59.4% reported being exposed to online hate in April and 58.7% reported seeing hate in November. Similarly, rates of exposure among American young adults remained stable (54.1% in April and 54.7% in November). Neither of these changes were statistically significant.[8] Thus, the increase in exposure observed in the United States was among those over the age of 25. Among those American respondents 26 or over, the percentage reporting seeing online hate increased from 33.0% to 39.2% between April and November. Among Finns this age, rates of exposure did not change.[9]

Consequently, rates of exposure to online hate increased as the pandemic unfolded; however, they only did so in the United States, and they only did so among Americans over the age of 25. What can account for the differences between the nations, and what can possibly account for the increase in exposure witnessed in the United States as the pandemic unfolded?

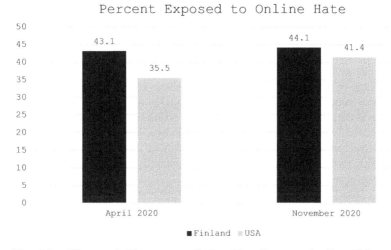

Fig. 6.3.   Changes in Exposure to Online Hate Between April and November 2020.

---

[7]The difference is not statistically significant ($\chi^2 = 2.43$; $p = 0.121$).
[8]The differences are not statistically significant (Finland: $\chi^2 = 0.02$; $p = 0.886$; the United States $\chi^2 = 0.01$; $p = 0.901$).
[9]The difference in the United States was statistically significant ($\chi^2 = 10.68$; $p < 0.001$). In Finland, rates of exposure went from 40.8% in April to 41.8% in November, which was not a significant change ($p = 0.591$).

## Accounting for the Cross-national Differences in Exposure to Hate During the Pandemic

To explain the cross-national differences, we first used a binary logistic regression model to see if common correlates of exposure held in both countries. Using age, sex, education, and if the respondents received their news primarily from online sources to predict exposure, we find that these factors relate to exposure as expected in both countries except for sex. The results are reported in Table 6.1.

In both countries, getting your news from online sources significantly increases exposure by 76% in Finland and 85% in the United States. Age decreases the likelihood of exposure in both nations (by 0.02% in both nations) and having a college degree significantly increases the likelihood of exposure (by 19% in Finland and 27% in the United States). All of these correlates appear to influence exposure similarly in both nations; however, sex is related to exposure only in Finland. In Finland, females are significantly more likely to report seeing online hate (34% more likely to see it than are Finnish males), but the effect is not statistically significant in the United States. As seen in the cross-tabular analysis presented above, the timing of data collection mattered in the United States but not in Finland. In the United States, respondents were 36% more likely to report seeing hate in November than they were in April, but this effect was not observed in Finland.

For our purposes, however, the focus is not really on what accounts for differences in exposure to online hate as there is already a sizable literature on this topic (Costello et al., 2016, 2020, 2021; Keipi et al., 2017, etc.). The point of this analysis is threefold. First, it demonstrates that the rates of exposure observed in these nations at these two times are related to predictors of exposure that have

Table 6.1. Logistic Regression of Exposure to Online Hate in Finland and the United States.

| | Finland | | | United States | | |
|---|---|---|---|---|---|---|
| | Coefficient | Standard Error | Odds Ratio | Coefficient | Standard Error | Odds Ratio |
| November 2020a | 0.054 | 0.074 | 1.055 | 0.309*** | 0.077 | 1.362 |
| Online news | 0.565*** | 0.093 | 1.759 | 0.613*** | 0.080 | 1.846 |
| Age | –0.022*** | 0.002 | .978 | –0.012*** | 0.002 | 0.988 |
| Female | 0.293*** | 0.075 | 1.341 | –0.046 | 0.077 | 0.955 |
| College degree | 0.175* | 0.076 | 1.191 | 0.237** | 0.079 | 1.267 |
| Constant | 0.040 | 0.139 | 1.041 | –0.538*** | 0.140 | 0.584 |

[a]November 2020 is compared to March 2020.
* $p < 0.05$; ** $p < 0.01$; *** $p < 0.001$.

## 96  James Hawdon

been reported by others. This gives us confidence that our data are measuring hate and its correlates similarly to those whose work came before us. Second, the analysis demonstrates that the changes in rates of exposure in the United States cannot be explained by factors commonly found to be correlated with exposure. Thus, the increase in exposure among Americans was not due to them getting news from online sources more frequently as the pandemic unfolded. This may have happened, but even if it did, this alone would not account for the increase in hate exposure since the effect is observed even while controlling for this factor. Third and most importantly, the analysis increases our confidence that over the course of the pandemic rates of exposure in the United States increased while they remained the same in Finland.

So, what can account for the difference? While our data cannot critically test this assertion, the likely difference between Finland and the United States was in how the pandemic was described and discussed by political leaders. Relying on other data, the increase in online hate and offline hate crime witnessed in the United States primarily targeted Asians as China and Chinese nationals were blamed for the pandemic (California Department of Justice, 2021; Gover et al., 2020; Lu & Sheng, 2020), and there is evidence that this increase was fueled by how then President Trump discussed the pandemic. His rhetoric was dramatically different from that of Finnish Prime Minister Marin, and this difference can help explain the cross-national difference in online hate exposure.

## President Trump's and Prime Minister Marin's COVID-19 Rhetoric and its Effect on Hate

The many curious statements by President Trump (e.g., injecting disinfectants inside the body at the site of a coronavirus infection to clean the lungs)[10] and missteps by his administration over the course of the pandemic are well documented. Indeed, some have estimated that approximately 40% of COVID-19-related deaths in the United States could have been prevented had the Trump administration acted like other G7 nations (Woolhandler et al., 2021). A large part of this story of curious statements involves the president's attempts to downplay the seriousness of the pandemic. For example, in early February 2020 when the virus first started to wreak havoc in the United States, President Trump asserted that the virus would "go away in April" (quoted in Wolfe & Dale, 2020). The president continued to assert that the pandemic would simply "go away" even as the cases started to mount. For example, on March 31, 2020, when the United States was

---

[10]Stories claiming President Trump recommended injecting bleach are inaccurate. What he said was: "I see the disinfectant that knocks it out in a minute, one minute. And is there a way we can do something like that by injection inside or almost a cleaning? As you see, it gets in the lungs, it does a tremendous number on the lungs, so it would be interesting to check that" (NBC News, 2020, April 24). Despite his suggestion, Homeland Security officials later confirmed that federal laboratories were not considering such a treatment option, according to NBC News.

*COVID-19 and the Flames of Hate* **97**

averaging 22,671 new cases each day, President Trump said, "it's going to go away, hopefully at the end of the month. And, if not, hopefully it will be soon after that" (as quoted in Wolfe & Dale, 2020). Indeed, President Trump was consistent in his use of this rhetoric of denial. Although he eventually focused on how the newly developed vaccines and therapeutics would make the virus "disappear," his downplaying of the threat the virus posed and its likely persistence never wavered (see the timeline by Wolfe & Dale, 2020).

Prime Minister Marin's rhetoric concerning the dangers posed by the pandemic differed dramatically from President Trump's. For example, in a press conference on February 27, 2020, Prime Minister Marin noted that, while the epidemic was rapidly spreading elsewhere, there was not an epidemic in Finland at the time. Yet, contrary to Trump's claims it would simply disappear, Marin also stressed that the government would remain vigilant. She also had the Minister of Social Affairs and Health Pekonen explain that the country had good preparedness and the masks in the country's stockpiles, while past the expiration date, could be used (Koljonen & Palonen, 2021). Although the discursive performances would evolve as the pandemic unfolded, the government's initial pandemic communication aimed to alleviate the public's concerns, communicate government actions, and provide scientifically informed health information about on the pandemic (see Koljonen & Palonen, 2021; Lindholm et al., 2023).

This rhetorical difference between the two nation's leaders had far-reaching consequences. Most importantly for our purposes, Trump's rhetoric of denial politicized and polarized a medical issue (see An et al., 2021; Piazza, 2020). In such a polarized atmosphere, the president faced increasing criticism of his administration that largely matched political lines. President Trump responded to this polarization and increased scrutiny in a manner that helped fan the flames of hate. As noted above and in contrast to Prime Minister Marin, President Trump attempted to downplay the seriousness of the virus. One way he did this was by praising China's President Xi's handling of the crises. For example, on February 25, 2020, President Trump said,

> China is working very, very hard. I have spoken to President Xi, and they're working very hard. And if you know anything about him, I think he'll be in pretty good shape. They're – they've had a rough patch, and I think right now they have it—it looks like they're getting it under control more and more. They're getting it more and more under control. So I think that's a problem that's going to go away.

Yet, unlike his rhetoric of denial that continued throughout the pandemic, his description of China's role in fighting the pandemic quickly changed. Less than a month after praising President Xi, President Trump referred to COVID-19 as "the Chinese virus" in a March 16th Tweet. He said, "The United States will be powerfully supporting those industries, like Airlines and others, that are particularly affected by the China Virus." After that initial Tweet, the president continued to refer to COVID-19 in terms related to China. Throughout 2020, President

## 98  *James Hawdon*

Trump referred to COVID-19 as "China flu," "China plague," "the China Virus," "Chinese plague," "Chinese flu," "Kung flu," and "Wuhan Virus" in various election rallies, press conferences, and Tweets (see Kurilla, 2021). He continued to describe the virus in these terms even after being questioned about the term being racist and xenophobic (Chakraborty, 2020; Vazequez & Klein, 2020). Yet, his anti-Chinese rhetoric intensified when, during a June rally in Tulsa, Oklahoma, he referred to the virus as "kung flu" (BBC News, 2020; Kurilla, 2021). Throughout his time in office, the president continued referring to COVID-19 in ways that directly connected it to China and the Chinese people.

President Trump also changed his rhetoric about how President Xi handled the initial stages of the pandemic. Just 6 months after praising Xi, President Trump blamed China for spreading COVID-19 and accused the Chinese government of misleading the world about the virus in a speech to the United Nations. During that speech, President Trump implied that China and the World Health Organization cooperated in covering up the danger of the pandemic. As quoted in Neuman (2020), President Trump said,

> The Chinese government and the World Health Organization – which is virtually controlled by China – falsely declared that there was no evidence of human-to-human transmission. Later, they falsely said people without symptoms would not spread the disease.

Trump also said, "In the earliest days of the virus, China locked down travel domestically while allowing flights to leave China and infect the world," and "China condemned my travel ban on their country, even as they canceled domestic flights and locked citizens in their homes" (quoted in Neuman, 2020). Therefore, not only did he use rhetoric that equated the virus with China, but he openly blamed China for the virus's deadly spread.

Again, Prime Minister Marin's discussion of the virus was starkly different from that of the American president. First, she avoided blaming China for the virus, and she never referred to the virus in ways that would link it to China or its citizens. In fact, this rhetoric of blame was apparently unique to President Trump. In a study of speeches made by 20 heads of government from around the world, Trump was the only leader to consistently refer to COVID-19 as "the Chinese virus" or the "China virus" (Dada et al., 2021). Prime Minister Marin always referred to the virus using its official name, as did the various government officials with whom she worked. Thus, Trump blamed China, thereby conflating the public health issue with politics, while Marin's rhetoric focused on the virus as a public health issue.

Trump's and Marin's rhetoric also differed in terms of the appeals to the public's emotions. President Trump openly blamed China for the virus, and he frequently used the rhetoric of war to make emotional appeals to the public. Of the 20 world leaders studied by Dada et al. (2021), male leaders were more likely to use a war metaphor than were female leaders. However, Trump invoked a war metaphor more often than any other leader, using war analogies 136 times in 23 speeches. To put that number in perspective, the leader who used war analogies the next most frequent was India's Prime Minister Narendra Modi. He made 30 references to war in his pandemic-related speeches. In contrast, Prime Minister Marian used a war analogy only once. Like other female world leaders, she was far more likely to use empathetic and personal appeals that focused on compassion and social cohesion (Dada et al., 2021; Lindholm et al., 2023). While both styles of appealing to the public are meant to generate emotions of unity, the rhetoric of war promotes collectivism based on fear, conflict, and division, while unity spawned by appeals to empathy are rooted in compassion and social cohesion (Ruiter et al., 2014). In fact, war metaphors are well known for "othering" and creating an "us vs. them" mentality.

Thus, the rhetoric used to describe the pandemic varied considerably between the two world leaders, and the effect of the rhetorical differences on hate is predictable. Several studies have documented how the spread of anti-Asian hate (in general) and anti-Chinese hate spread online following Trump's Tweets and speeches. For example, analyzing Tweets 1 week before and 1 week following the president's first "China Virus" Tweet, Hswen et al. (2021) found that hashtags that included #chinesevirus were more than twice as likely to contain anti-Asian hate than did those that referenced the virus as #Covid19. Moreover, when the week before the first Tweet is compared to the week that followed it, the use of hashtags with #chinesevirus significantly increased compared with hashtags including #Covid19 (Hswen et al., 2021). Costello et al. (2021) also found that Tweets containing inflammatory language surged immediately following the former-president's use of "China Virus." Kim and Kesari (2021) also found that Trump's anti-Asian speech increased the prevalence of anti-Asian hate speech, counterhate speech, and the spread of misinformation in the 59,337 Tweets related to COVID-19 they analyzed. Indeed, the online anti-Asian hate spread quickly and seemed to be normalized over the course of the pandemic (see Costello et al., 2021), as after the president referred to the virus as the "China virus," several other government officials began to describe the coronavirus in a similar fashion and aggressively blame China for the pandemic (Rogers, 2020; Wu, 2020). Given the surge in online anti-Asian hate speech following the President's rhetoric directly associating the coronavirus with China and his administrations' continued use of such rhetoric, it is unsurprising that more Americans saw online hate in November 2020 than saw it in April 2020.

# Conclusion: Online Hate Exposure, Political Rhetoric, and Policy Implications

The policy implications of our findings in this chapter are clear. As documented here, exposure to online hate increased significantly in the United States between the onset of the pandemic and eight months later. This increase was not seen in Finland. While we cannot say conclusively that it was the rhetoric President Trump used to describe COVID-19 that caused this increase, there is ample evidence that his referencing the virus as the "China virus," "Chinese virus," and "Kung flu" led to a barrage of anti-Chinese online discourse. It logically follows that this contributed to more Americans seeing online hate in November 2020 than in

## 100  James Hawdon

March 2020. Given the stark contrast between the president's rhetoric and Prime Minister Marin's, we are confident that this difference at least contributed to the different trajectories of hate seen in the two nations as the pandemic unfolded. Assuming this argument is correct, the heightened exposure to online hate in the United States likely had consequences. As documented above, it likely contributed to the increase in anti-Asian hate crime witnessed in the United States during the pandemic. While hate crimes increased in both the United States and Finland during the pandemic, the increase was more pronounced in the United States. Moreover, the increase in hate crimes in the United States was particularly targeting Asians, who were also the targets of President Trump's anti-Chinese rhetoric around COVID-19 and the online hate that followed his speeches and Tweets. In fact, comparing 2019 to 2020, anti-Asian hate crimes increased by 145% in America's largest cities while overall hate crime decreased by 6% in those cities (Center for the Study of Hate and Extremism, 2021).[11] This is unlikely to be a coincidence.

Another likely consequence of increased exposure to online hate is its effect on citizens' perceptions of the government, social institutions, and their fellow citizens. Hate creates "us" and "them," which in turn sows division and polarization. Given that much of the hate seen online today is rightwing hate that promotes cynicism toward and mistrust of the government, exposure to online hate can undermine compliance with government-issued health recommendations (Bish & Michie, 2010; Choi & Fox, 2022; Doogan et al., 2020; Kestilä-Kekkonen et al., 2022; Sedgwick et al., 2022). Given that complying with these recommendations saved lives (e.g., Howard et al., 2021; Miyazawa & Kaneko, 2020; Motallebi et al., 2022), widespread exposure to hate can indirectly increase the severity of COVID-19 by decreasing compliance with health-protective behaviors. This explicit connection between hate exposure and compliance will be explored in later chapters. For now, however, this chapter highlights the ability of politicians and policymakers to steer social media narratives and influence the broader public discourse. When these individuals help create a narrative of hate, more people will likely be exposed to it. Consequences that follow this heightened exposure are unfortunate but predictable.

## References

Allen, J. M., & Norris, G. H. (2011). Is genocide different? Dealing with hate speech in a post-genocide society. *Journal of International Law and International Relations, 7*, 146–174.

An, J., Kwak, H., Lee, C. S., Jun, B., & Ahn, Y. Y. (2021). *Predicting anti-Asian hateful users on Twitter during COVID-19.* arXiv preprint arXiv:2109.07296

BBC News. (2020). *President Trump calls coronavirus 'kung flu'.* https://www.bbc.com/news/av/world-us-canada-53173436

---

[11]See Koski and Bantley (2020) for a general argument of how the Trump's administration influenced hate crimes.

Bish, A., & Michie, S. (2010). Demographic and attitudinal determinants of protective behaviours during a pandemic: A review. *British Journal of Health Psychology, 15,* 797–824.

Blazak, R. (2009). Toward a working definition of hate groups. In B. Perry, B. Levin, P. Iganski, R. Blazak, & F. Lawrence (Eds.), *Hate crimes* (pp. 133–148). Greenwood Publishing Group.

Bleich, E. (2011). The rise of Hate Bowman-Grieve, Lorraine. 2009. Exploring 'Stormfront': A virtual community of the radical right. *Studies in Conflict & Terrorism, 32*(11), 989–1007.

Bowman-Grieve, L. (2009). Exploring "Stormfront": A virtual community of the radical right. *Studies in Conflict & Terrorism, 32*(11), 989–1007.

California Department of Justice. (2021). *Anti-Asian hate crime events during the COVID-19 pandemic.* California Department of Justice Research Center. https://oag.ca.gov/system/files/media/anti-asian-hc-report.pdf

Center for the Study of Hate and Extremism. (2021). *Fact sheet: Anti-Asian hate crime reported to police in America's largest cities: 2019 & 2020.* https://www.csusb.edu/sites/default/files/FACT%20SHEET-%20Anti-Asian%20Hate%202020%20rev%203.21.21.pdf

Chakraborty, B. (2020). Trump doubles down on "China virus;" Demands to know who in White House used phrase Kung Flu. *Fox News.* https://www.foxnews.com/politics/trump-coronavirus-china-virus-white-house-kung-flu

Chan, J., Ghose, A., & Seamans, R. (2016). The internet and racial hate crime. Mis Quarterly, *40*(2), 381–404.

Choi, Y., & Fox, A. M. (2022). Mistrust in public health institutions is a stronger predictor of vaccine hesitancy and uptake than trust in Trump. *Social Science & Medicine, 314,* 115440.

Cohen, L. E., & Felson, M. (1979). Social change and crime rate trends: A routine activity approach. *American Sociological Review, 44,* 588–608.

Costello, M., Barret-Fox, R., Bernatzky, C., Hawdon, J., & Mendes, K. (2020). Predictors of viewing online extremism among America's youth. *Youth & Society, 52*(5), 710–727.

Costello, M., Cheng, L., Luo, F., Hu, H., Liao, S., Vishwamitra, N., Li, M., & Okpala, E. (2021). COVID-19: A pandemic of anti-Asian cyberhate. *Journal of Hate Studies, 17*(1), 108–118.

Costello, M., & Hawdon, J. (2020). Hate speech in online spaces. In A. Bossler & T. Holt (Eds.), *The Palgrave handbook of international cybercrime and cyberdeviance* (pp. 1397–1416). Palgrave. https://doi.org/10.1007/978-3-319-78440-3_60

Costello, M., Hawdon, J., Ratliff, T., & Grantham, T. (2016). Who views online extremism? Individual attributes leading to exposure. *Computers in Human Behavior, 63,* 311–320.

Costello, M., Restifo, S. J., & Hawdon, J. (2021). Viewing anti-immigrant hate online: An application of routine activity and social structure social learning theory. *Computers in Human Behavior, 124.* https://doi.org/10.1016/j.chb.2021.106927.

Costello, M., Rukus, J., & Hawdon, J. (2019). We don't like your type around here: Regional and residential differences in exposure to online hate material targeting sexuality. *Deviant Behavior, 40*(3), 385–401.

Dada, S., Ashworth, H. C., Bewa, M. J., & Dhatt, R. (2021). Words matter: Political and gender analysis of speeches made by heads of government during the COVID-19 pandemic. *BMJ Global Health, 6*(1), e003910.

Doogan, C., Buntine, W., Linger, H., & Brunt, S. (2020). Public perceptions and attitudes toward COVID-19 nonpharmaceutical interventions across six countries: A topic modeling analysis of Twitter data. *Journal of medical Internet research, 22*(9), e21419.

## 102 James Hawdon

Federal Bureau of Investigation (FBI). (2011). *Domestic terrorism: Focus on militia extremism.* https://www.fbi.gov/news/stories/2011/september/militia_092211

Foxman, A. H., & Wolf, C. (2013). *Viral hate: Containing its spread on the internet.* Macmillan.

Freilich, J., Belli, R., & Chermak, S. (2011). *United States extremist crime database (ECDB) 1990–2010.* http://www.start.umd.edu/research-projects/united-states-extremist-crime-database-ecdb-1990-2010

Gartner. (2020, March 19). *Gartner HR survey reveals 88% of organizations have encouraged or required employees to work from home due to coronavirus.* Gartner. Retrieved May 3, 2020, from https://www.gartner.com/en/newsroom/press-releases/2020-03-19-gartner-hr-survey-reveals-88%2D%2Dof-organizationshave-e

Gover, A. R., Harper, S. B., & Langton, L. (2020). Anti-Asian hate crime during the COVID-19 pandemic: Exploring the reproduction of inequality. *American Journal of Criminal Justice, 45,* 647–667.

Hawdon, J. (2012). Applying differential association theory to online hate groups: A theoretical statement. *Journal of Research on Finnish Society, 5,* 39–47.

Hawdon, J., Bernatzky, C., & Costello, M. (2019). Cyber-routines, political attitudes, and exposure to violence-advocating online extremism. *Social Forces, 98*(1), 329–354.

Hawdon, J., Oksanen, A., & Räsänen, P. (2014). Victims of online hate groups: American youth's exposure to online hate speech. In J. Hawdon, J. Ryan, & M. Lucht (Eds.), *The causes and consequences of group violence: From bullies to terrorists* (pp. 165–182). Lexington Books.

Hawdon, J., Oksanen, A., & Räsänen, P. (2015). Online extremism and online hate: Exposure among adolescents and young adults in four nations. *Nordicom-Information, 37,* 29–37.

Hawdon, J., Oksanen, A. & Räsänen, P. (2017). Exposure to online hate in four nations: A cross-national consideration. *Deviant Behavior, 38*(3), 254–266.

Hawdon, J., Parti, K., & Dearden, T. E. (2020). Cybercrime in America amid COVID-19: The initial results from a natural experiment. *American Journal of Criminal Justice, 45*(4), 546–562.

Hawdon, J., Reichelmann, A., & Costello, M. (2022). Riding the cyberwaves: The ebbs and flows of Internet cyberhate. In R. Baikady, S. Sajid, V. Nadesan, J. Przeperski, M. R. Islam, & J. Gao (Eds.), *The Palgrave handbook of global social change* (pp. 1–15). Palgrave Macmillan. https://doi.org/10.1007/978-3-030-87624-1_296-1

Holt, T. J., Freilich, J. D., Chermak, S. M., Mills, C., & Silva, J. (2019). Loners, colleagues, or peers? Assessing the social organization of radicalization. *American Journal of Criminal Justice, 44*(1), 83–105.

Howard, J., Huang, A., Li, Z., Tufekci, Z., Zdimal, V., van der Westhuizen, H. M., & Rimoin, A. W. (2021). An evidence review of face masks against COVID-19. *Proceedings of the National Academy of Sciences, 118*(4), e2014564118.

Hswen, Y., Xu, X., Hing, A., Hawkins, J. B., Brownstein, J. S., & Gee, G. C. (2021). Association of "# covid19" versus "# chinesevirus" with anti-Asian sentiments on Twitter: March 9–23, 2020. *American Journal of Public Health, 111*(5), 956–964.

Keipi, T., Näsi, M., Oksanen, A., & Räsänen, P. (2017). *Online hate and harmful content: Cross-national perspectives.* Routledge.

Keipi, T., Räsänen, P., Oksanen, A., Hawdon, J., & Näsi, M. (2017). Harm-advocating online content and subjective well-being: A cross-national study of new risks faced by youth. *Journal of Risk Research, 20*(3), 634–649.

Kestilä-Kekkonen, E., Koivula, A., & Tiihonen, A. (2022). When trust is not enough. A longitudinal analysis of political trust and political competence during the first wave of the COVID-19 pandemic in Finland. *European Political Science Review, 14*(3), 424–440.

Kim, J. Y., & Kesari, A. (2021). Misinformation and hate speech: The case of anti-Asian hate speech during the COVID-19 pandemic. *Journal of Online Trust and Safety, 1*(1), 1–14.

## COVID-19 and the Flames of Hate 103

Koljonen, J., & Palonen, E. (2021). Performing COVID-19 control in Finland: Interpretative topic modelling and discourse theoretical reading of the government communication and hashtag landscape. *Frontiers in Political Science, 3*, 689614.

Koski, S. V., & Bantley, K. (2020). Dog whistle politics: The Trump administration's influence on hate crimes. *Seton Hall Legislative Journal, 44*, 39–60.

Kurilla, R. (2021). "Kung Flu" – The dynamics of fear, popular culture, and authenticity in the anatomy of populist communication. Frontiers in Communication, *6*, 624643.

Lake, D. A., & Rothchild, D. (1998). *The international spread of ethnic conflict: Fear, diffusion, and escalation*. Princeton University Press.

Lindholm, J., Carlsson, T., Albrecht, F., & Hermansson, H. (2023). Communicating Covid-19 on social media: Analysing the use of Twitter and Instagram by Nordic health authorities and prime ministers. In B. Johansson, Ø. Ihlen, J. Lindholm, & M. Blach-Ørsten (Eds.), *Communicating a pandemic: Crisis management and Covid-19 in the Nordic countries* (pp. 149–172). University of Gothenburg. https://doi.org/10.48335/9789188855688-7

Lu, R., & Sheng, Y. (2020). *From fear to hate: How the COVID-19 pandemic sparks racial animus in the United States*. arXiv preprint arXiv:2007.01448.

McCaulley, C. (2016). *Terrorism research and public policy*. Routledge.

Ministry of Justice Finland. (2012). *Criminal code*. Retrieved November 16, 2014, from www.finlex.fi/fi/laki/kaannokset/1889/en18890039

Miyazawa, D., & Kaneko, G. (2020). *Face mask wearing rate predicts country's COVID-19 death rates*. medRxiv.

Motallebi, S., Cheung, R. C., Mohit, B., Shahabi, S., Tabriz, A. A., & Moattari, S. (2022). Modeling COVID-19 mortality across 44 countries: Face covering may reduce deaths. *American Journal of Preventive Medicine, 62*(4), 483–491.

Müller, K., & Schwarz, C. (2021). Fanning the flames of hate: Social media and hate crime. *Journal of the European Economic Association, 19*(4), 2131–2167.

NBC News. (2020, April 24). *Trump suggests 'injection' of disinfectant to beat coronavirus and 'clean' the lungs*. https://www.nbcnews.com/politics/donald-trump/trump-suggests-injection-disinfectant-beat-coronavirus-clean-lungs-n1191216

Näsi, M., Räsänen, P., Hawdon, J., Holkeri, E., & Oksanen, A. (2015). Exposure to online hate material and social trust among Finnish youth. *Information, Technology and People, 28*(3), 607–622.

Neuman, S. (2020). *In UN speech, Trump blasts China and WHO, blaming them for spread of COVID-19*. NPR. https://www.npr.org/sections/coronavirus-live-updates/2020/09/22/915630892/in-u-n-speech-trump-blasts-china-and-who-blaming-them-for-spread-of-covid-19

OSCE. (2022). Organization for security and co-operation in Europe. Hate Crime Reporting: Finland. https://hatecrime.osce.org/finland

Phadke, S., Lloyd, J., Hawdon, J., Samory, M., & Mitra, T. (2018). Framing hate with hate frames: Designing the codebook. In *Companion of the 2018 ACM conference on computer supported cooperative work and social computing* (pp. 201–204). ACM. https://doi.org/10.1145/3272973.3274055

Piazza, J. A. (2020). Politician hate speech and domestic terrorism. *International Interactions, 46*(3), 431–453.

Pariser, E. (2011). *The filter bubble: What the Internet is hiding from you*. Penguin.

Potok, M. (2015). *The year in hate and extremism. Intelligence report: 141*. https://www.splcenter.org/fighting-hate/intelligence-report/2015/year-hate-and-extremism-0

Reichelmann, A., Hawdon, J., Costello, M., Ryan, J., Blaya, C., Llorent, V., Oksanen, A., Räsänen, P., & Zych, I. (2021). Hate knows no boundaries: Online hate in six nations. *Deviant Behavior, 42*(9), 1100–1111. https://doi.org/10.1080/01639625.2020.1722337

Rogers, K. (2020, March 10). Politicians' use of 'Wuhan virus' starts a debate health experts wanted to avoid. *The New York Times*. https://www.nytimes.com/2020/03/10/us/politics/wuhan-virus.html

## 104    James Hawdon

Ruiter, R. A., Kessels, L. T., Peters, G. J. Y., & Kok, G. (2014). Sixty years of fear appeal research: Current state of the evidence. *International Journal of Psychology, 49*(2), 63–70.

Sedgwick, D., Hawdon, J., Räsänen, P., & Koivula, A. (2022). The role of collaboration in complying with Covid-19 health protective behaviors: A cross-national study. *Administration & Society, 54*(1), 29–56.

Shapiro, J. L. (2016). We hate what we fear: Interpersonal hate from a clinical perspective. In K. Aumer (Ed.), *The psychology of love and hate in intimate relationships* (pp. 153–177). Springer.

Snow, D., Tan, A. & Owens, P. (2013). Social movements, framing processes, and cultural revitalization and fabrication. Mobilization: An International Quarterly, *18*(3), 225–242.

Soral, W., Bilewicz, M., & Winiewski, M. (2018). Exposure to hate speech increases prejudice through desensitization. *Aggressive Behavior, 44*(2), 136–146.

Southern Poverty Law Center. (2017). *Extremist files.* https://www.splcenter.org/fighting-hate/extremist-files

Southern Poverty Law Center. (2022). *Antigovernment movement.* https://www.splcenter.org/fighting-hate/extremist-files/ideology/antigovernment

Sternberg, R. J. (2020). FLOTSAM: A theory of the development and transmission of hate. In R. J. Sternberg (Ed.), *Perspectives on hate: How it originates, develops, manifests, and spreads* (pp. 3–24). American Psychological Association. https://doi.org/10.1037/0000180-001

Suny, R. G. (2004). *Why we hate you: The passions of national identity and ethnic violence.* https://escholarship.org/content/qt3pv4g8zf/qt3pv4g8zf.pdf

The New America Foundation International Security Program. (2015). *Homegrown extremists.* http://securitydata.newamerica.net/extremists/deadly-attacks.html

Tynes, B. (2006). Children, adolescents, and the culture of hate online. In N. Dowd, D. Singer, & R. F. Wilson (Eds.), *Handbook of children, culture, and violence* (pp. 267–289). Sage.

US Department of Justice. (2020). *Hate crime statistics.* US Department of Justice. https://www.justice.gov/crs/highlights/2020-hate-crimes-statistics

US Department of Justice. (2021). *Hate crime statistics.* US Department of Justice. https://www.justice.gov/hatecrimes/hate-crime-statistics

Vazequez, M., & Klein, B. (2020). *Trump again defends use of the term "China Virus.* CNNpolitics. https://www.cnn.com/2020/03/17/politics/trump-china-coronavirus/index.html

Wolfe, D., & Dale, D. (2020, October 31). *It's going to disappear: A timeline of Trump's claims that Covid-19 will vanish.* CNN. https://www.cnn.com/interactive/2020/10/politics/covid-disappearing-trump-comment-tracker/

Woolhandler, S., Himmelstein, D. U., Ahmed, S., Bailey, Z., Bassett, M. T., Bird, M., Bor, J., Bor, D., Carrasquillo, O., Chowkwanyun, M., & Dickman, S. L. (2021). Public policy and health in the Trump era. *The Lancet, 397*(10275), 705–753.

Wu, N. (2020, March 18). USA Today: GOP senator says China 'to blame' for coronavirus spread because of 'culture where people eat bats and snakes and dogs'. *USA Today.* https://www.usatoday.com/story/news/politics/2020/03/18/coronavirus-sen-john-cornyn-says-chinese-eating-bats-spread-virus/2869342001/

Section 3

# COVID-19 and the Public: Well-being, Compliance, and Health Outcomes

Chapter 7

# Coping, Well-being, and COVID-19

*Donna Sedgwick*

*Virginia Tech, USA*

## Abstract

This chapter examines which coping mechanisms citizens used during the pandemic and how these mechanisms related to overall well-being. Using the Transaction Theory of Stress and Coping to frame the analysis, the chapter investigates predictive factors for various coping strategies and identifies which groups were more likely to use adaptive as opposed to maladaptive strategies. I examine how coping strategies used in April 2020 predict change in well-being, measured by life satisfaction, in November 2020. Americans reported greater use of maladaptive coping and less use of the adaptive coping strategies compared to their Finnish counterparts. Americans reported more frequent use of religious coping strategies. Interestingly, worrying about COVID-19 did not increase the use of maladaptive coping for Finns or Americans. Regarding the effect of the coping strategies on life satisfaction, the analyses revealed that those who reported using maladaptive strategies in April 2020 showed a significant decrease in life satisfaction in November 2020. However, this finding was only significant for Finnish residents. Unexpectedly, Finnish and US residents who reported using Active/Expressive and Planning coping reported a decrease in life satisfaction from April to November 2020. Finally, Finnish and US residents who were married, had higher self-esteem, or had higher social capital were more likely to report an increase in life satisfaction from April 2020 to November 2020. These findings raise questions for future research. The context of the pandemic may have created a unique situation that rendered coping mechanisms to behave in unusual ways.

*Keywords*: Coping strategies; well-being; the Transaction Theory of Stress and Coping; mental health; COVID-19 as stressor

---

Perceptions of a Pandemic: A Cross-Continental Comparison of Citizen Perceptions, Attitudes, and Behaviors During COVID-19, 107–124

Copyright © 2025 by Donna Sedgwick

Published under exclusive licence by Emerald Publishing Limited

doi:10.1108/978-1-83608-624-620241007

## 108  *Donna Sedgwick*

## Introduction

The COVID-19 pandemic affected many aspects of life, including work and industry, educational institutions, family dynamics, leisure and social networks, and healthcare systems. However, experts also raised concerns about the impact of COVID-19 on personal mental health and well-being. Scholars argued that the pandemic had the potential to exacerbate mental health issues and decrease well-being due to having characteristics of a traumatic or stressful event (Horesh & Brown, 2020; Shamblaw et al., 2021). Additionally, the stay-at-home and social distancing orders put in place decreased the likelihood of people seeking solace and comfort in face-to-face interactions with their extended family and social networks, which also affected mental health and quality of life factors (Agha, 2021; Clair et al., 2021; Vos, 2021). Indeed, the World Health Organization expressed that the mental health concerns resulting from the pandemic were some of the most pressing issues for consideration (World Health Organization, 2022). Psychologists and others have long posited that when people are presented with stressors and traumatic events, they interpret those stressors and respond with varying types of coping strategies (Lazarus & Folkman, 1984).

With the major life event that the pandemic presented for people between March 2020 and December 2020, it is valuable to understand how coping varied and how various coping strategies affected overall well-being. Additionally, research has suggested that people used coping strategies more often in the earlier stages of the pandemic compared to the later stages (Lueger-Schuster et al., 2022; Meyer et al., 2022). This chapter investigates the various factors that affected coping and well-being within the first eight months of the pandemic.

Similar to a war or natural disaster, scholars argue that the COVID-19 pandemic shares characteristics of a traumatic or stressful life event (Horesh & Brown, 2020; Shamblaw et al., 2021). Stressful life events have the potential for creating threats or challenges in peoples' lives (Chen et al., 2022). Characteristics of stressful life events include the potential for direct impact on an individual or their family, the lack of control an individual has in controlling the event, and the severity of the perceived event (Jean-Baptiste et al., 2020; Peacock & Wong, 1990). Early in the COVID-19 pandemic when transmission of the disease was still largely unknown and the death toll began rising quickly, it is evident that the pandemic met these criteria. Additionally, scholars discuss secondary stressors that occur with stressful life events, such as negative impacts on individuals' financial situations or disruptions like schools and places of employment shutting down and turning to remote modalities (Coiro et al., 2021; Maestripieri, 2021; Rogowska et al., 2021; Vos, 2021). These secondary stressors also correlate with higher levels of mental health issues, like depression and anxiety (Coiro et al., 2021). However, how all these stressors affect well-being and quality of life depends upon how individuals perceive them and the coping strategies people undertake to manage those stressors.

The TTSC (Lazarus & Folkman, 1984) posits that variation in how people respond to stressors is based upon differences in a primary appraisal of the stressor (i.e., assessing the characteristics of it discussed above) and a secondary appraisal that includes what, if any, actions or approaches they can take to handle the stressor. These appraisals result in coping strategies that are often broadly characterized in terms of their positive characteristics (adaptive coping) or negative characteristics (maladaptive coping), and whether the strategy is direct and action-based, or indirect and emotion-based. For example, an example of a positive direct coping strategy is seeking comfort from family or friends whereas an example of a negative direct coping strategy is seeking comfort from substance use.

Conversely, a positive indirect coping strategy could be the person reframing the stressor in a positive light, whereas a negative indirect coping strategy could the person blaming themselves for the stressor. While these examples suggest coping is positive, negative, direct, or indirect, many of the coping strategies fall along a continuum. For example, some other coping strategies include developing plans, venting, or using religion for comfort, which arguably are not as clearly defined as positive, negative, direct, or indirect. Why people choose the various coping strategies they do is not always straightforward; thus, it is valuable to understand what factors likely predict their use. Particularly during a stressful life event like the pandemic, identifying these factors can aid public and mental health professionals when trying to assess who uses what types of coping strategies and how successfully they adapt to the stressful situation.

## Factors That Affect Coping

Factors that affect coping can be generally grouped into four categories: demographic and internal personal/trait characteristics, interpersonal resources, contextual surroundings, and characteristics of the stressor itself. Given the focus of this book is on the COVID-19 pandemic and the characteristics of the stressor are held constant, I will not focus on how different stressors can result in varying coping mechanisms. However, it is important to note that researchers have identified many people responded to the pandemic with varying levels of stress (Wang et al., 2020).

Regarding demographic characteristics, findings often support that men and women use different coping strategies, particularly during the pandemic (Fluharty & Fancourt, 2021). Gender differences have been found in the perception of risk or uncertainty associated with the pandemic, although the direction has not been consistent in findings (Alaszewski, 2023; Chen et al., 2022; Huy, 2021; Snel et al., 2022). Some additional differences include women using more religious and denial coping compared to men, who used more active coping (Agha, 2021). However, women reported using some direct coping strategies more than men, such as social media use and mind–body practice (Krase et al., 2022).

Other demographic factors that affect coping include age, educational level, marital status, and religion. Generally speaking, older, educated, married persons report using more adaptive coping strategies (Filindassi et al., 2022; Javed & Parveen, 2021; Maestripieri, 2021; Meyer et al., 2022; Munsell et al., 2020; Snel et al., 2022). While not much research has focused specifically on religion as a factor determining assessment of risk and choice of coping strategy, David et al.'s (2022) systematic review of religion and coping find mixed results in how

# 110    Donna Sedgwick

religiosity affects assessment of COVID-19 risk. That is, studies find that religiosity both increases and decreases perceived risk. Regarding coping strategies, Javed and Parveen (2021) find that compared to Hindus and other religious groups, Muslims are more likely to use "escape" and "trust in God" coping strategies.

In addition to demographic characteristics, other individual factors, such as personal traits, viewpoints, and mental health conditions, have been investigated for their effects on coping. For example, Partouche-Sebban et al. (2021) identify that trust in institutions mediated the relationship between fear of death and the use of maladaptive coping during COVID-19, with those reporting increased fear of death being more likely to report higher institutional trust, and those with higher trust more likely to report using maladaptive behaviors. Conversely, increased self-esteem has been shown to correlate with an increase in the use of adaptive coping strategies (Schillinger & Stalpers, 2021). Additionally, pre-existing mental health conditions have also been found to affect possible coping strategies. For example, Fallahi et al. (2021) find that those persons with pre-existing psychiatric disorders are more likely to use maladaptive coping behaviors during COVID-19 compared to those without pre-existing disorders.

Along with internal characteristics affecting coping, scholars have found that national context also affects the perception of stress and the type of coping strategies used. For example, various comparative studies conducted during the pandemic have consistently found international differences in stress and well-being levels during the COVID-19 pandemic (Kirby et al., 2022; Mohamed et al., 2022). Additionally, Denisse et al. (2020) find that the use of religious coping and mental disengagement varied substantially based upon the country of the people surveyed.

Interpersonal resources, such as social relationships, consistently affect the selection of coping techniques. For example, social capital and social connectedness have been reported to matter for both primary and secondary appraisals of the stressors. Snel et al. (2022) and Jean-Baptiste et al. (2020) report that people with higher levels of social capital reported lower levels of stress and anxiety during COVID-19, and while not conducted during the pandemic, Wilczyńska et al. (2015) identify that people with stronger social belonging are less likely to engage in negative coping strategies when faced with a stressor. Conversely, those people reporting higher social isolation during the pandemic are more likely to report using substance use as a coping strategy (Clair et al., 2021). Thus, environmental context and interpersonal resources, like connections, also shape coping strategies.

## *Anticipate Findings*

Based upon prior TTSC research, I expect that older, married, and higher educated persons will report using more adaptive coping strategies than younger, single, and those with less education. I expect to find gender differences, although the direction is unclear. In addition, I expect to find a positive relationship between social capital and the use of adaptive coping strategies, and I expect to find a positive relationship between trust in science and maladaptive coping. Finally, I expect to find differences between US and Finnish citizens' use of various coping strategies, in particular for the use of religion coping.

## Analyzing the Predictors of Coping Strategies

To examine the coping strategies, I factor analyzed 27 measures of the BRIEF Cope (Carver, 1997). BRIEF Cope is a commonly used inventory to assess different types of coping strategies that includes indirect and direct adaptive and maladaptive coping approaches. The literature supports that the BRIEF Cope can vary in factor loading based upon the context and survey used (Solberg et al., 2022). I originally used a three-factor approach; however, based upon the literature that indicated that religion coping is a unique type of coping that produces outcomes different than perhaps would be expected (David et al., 2022), I forced the two religion coping measures into its own fourth factor. The other 25 measures loaded on three factors that I named maladaptive coping, active/expressive and planning coping, and positive reframing (see the Appendix for details about factor loadings for measures). I consider both the active/expressive and planning coping, and the positive reframing coping to be adaptive coping strategies, even though "saying unpleasant feelings" and "expressing negative feelings" are also included in the "active/expressive and planning" factor.

Using the factor loading scores, I ran each of the coping strategy factors as its own dependent variable and included various predictor variables to identify who is more likely to use the different coping strategies. I ran the analyses separately for the US and Finnish samples. The forest plots represent the betas for each factor and their 95% confidence intervals.

First, I investigated who is likely to use maladaptive coping (see Fig. 7.1).

Several significant predictors emerged when running a regression analysis to identify predictors of maladaptive coping during the early phase of the COVID-19

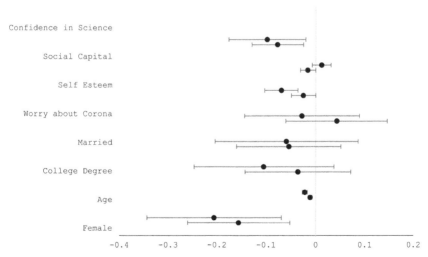

Fig. 7.1. Factors That Affect Maladaptive Coping: The United States and Finland. *Note*: US confidence intervals are presented as the top line in chart. US RSQ = 0.119, Finnish RSQ = 0.115.

## 112    Donna Sedgwick

pandemic. First, while not depicted in the displayed figures, I did run a regression with the entire sample, and US citizens were more likely than Finnish citizens to report using maladaptive coping. To continue the analysis, I separated the samples by country, and not surprisingly, found differences by country in the emergence of significant predictors. For Finnish residents, a few demographic/personal trait factors reduced the likelihood of using maladaptive coping, including being older, female, and having higher self-esteem. Additionally, those Finnish residents who reported having higher social capital and higher confidence in science were significantly less likely to use maladaptive coping. Comparatively, fewer predictors gained significance for US residents, although some similarities did emerge. Being older, female, and having higher self-esteem also reduced the likelihood of using maladaptive coping for the United States. Also, those US residents with greater confidence in science were less likely to use maladaptive coping. However, social capital was not a significant predictor in the United States. Across both counties, marital status, worrying about corona, or being college educated did not predict maladaptive coping. For both countries, a person's age had the strongest effect.

The analysis revealed some expected predictive factors – older persons, females, and those with higher self-esteem reported less use of maladaptive behaviors; additionally, I found differences by country. I also found some unexpected findings based upon the literature. While social capital has been reported to reduce the use of maladaptive behaviors (Fluharty & Fancourt, 2021; Wilczyńska et al., 2015), these findings suggest that only in Finland were those people with higher social capital less likely to engage in maladaptive coping behaviors. In fact, while not significant, in the United States the direction of social capital was trending toward positively influencing maladaptive behavior; that is, US residents with higher social capital were more likely to report maladaptive behaviors. As studies found that alcohol sales in the United States statistically increased between 2019 and 2020 (Lee et al., 2021), perhaps it is not surprising that people with higher social capital were partaking in alcohol use as a coping mechanism during these unprecedented times. Given the context of the pandemic being a new experience being undertaken by everyone, it is possible that the stigma normally assigned to selecting "I've been using alcohol or other drugs …" to "make myself feel better" or "to help me get through it" was lessened. In simple terms, people may have been gathering in their "small pod" with friends and family and partaking in alcohol to cope with the pandemic, particularly in the national context of the United States, which is arguably a "wet" culture (Seid et al., 2016).

Additionally, while Partouche-Sebban et al. (2021) found that trust in institutions led to an increase in maladaptive behaviors, I found the opposite finding for both countries. They based their argument that placing trust externally increased the likelihood of participating in maladaptive behaviors. However, our findings indicated that specifically having confidence in science could reduce these behaviors. Their study pulled out a specific segment of the population – those who reported increased fear of dying due to COVID-19 – so perhaps this can explain the difference. It could be that having trust in science helped alleviate fear about COVID-19, which in turn reduced the use of these maladaptive behaviors.

Next, I investigated predictors of active/expressive and planning coping (see Fig. 7.2).

*Coping, Well-being, and COVID-19* 113

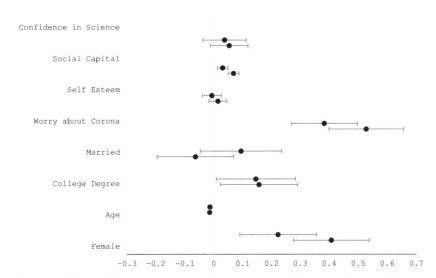

Fig. 7.2. Factors That Affect Active/Expressive and Planning Coping: The United States and Finland. *Note*: US confidence intervals are presented as the top line for each predictor. US RSQ = 0.148, Finnish RSQ = 0.245.

While the regression analysis of the entire sample revealed significant differences by country, with US residents reporting less use of active/expressive and planning coping compared to their Finnish counterparts, a similar set of predictor variables emerged for both countries. Moreover, predictors of active/expressive and planning coping yielded different results than for maladaptive coping. Females and those with college degrees were more likely to use active, expressive, or planning coping strategies. Additionally, those who reported higher social capital and worry about the Corona virus were also more likely to use these types of strategies. Worry about Coronavirus was the strongest positive predictor for both countries. In both Finland and the United States, being older significantly decreased the likelihood of using active, expressive, and planning coping. Being married, along with a person's confidence in science and self-esteem were unrelated to active/expressive and planning coping.

While finding that older persons were less likely to use active/expressing and planning coping is unexpected, some studies have found a null effect between age and adaptive coping behaviors (Meyer et al., 2022). What has been more readily found is that older persons are less likely to use maladaptive behaviors, and as discussed above, the results support this finding. Those with higher social capital and a college education were more likely to use expressive, planning, or problem-based methods, which is supported by previous literature also (Fluharty & Fancourt, 2021; Jean-Baptiste et al., 2020). Additionally, as worrying about a situation has been found to prompt engagement in social support and planning strategies in prior studies (Fluharty & Fancourt, 2021), it is not surprising that worrying about COVID-19 was positively associated with this coping approach.

Interestingly, while the stereotype of Americans is of a more expressive culture than the Finns, our findings support that they were less likely to use this coping strategy than their Finnish counterparts. This finding warrants further investigation.

Next, I examined the predictors for positive reframing coping (see Fig. 7.3).

Not as many significant factors emerged as predictors for positive reframing with some notable exceptions. Those people who reported higher self-esteem and confidence in science were more likely to use positive reframing coping strategies for both countries. Similar to the previous analysis, country differences emerged in the overall use of positive reframing, with US citizens using this coping strategy less. For both countries, confidence in science was the strongest predictor.

I point out that primarily the only significant factors for predicting positive reframing were individual perceptions and beliefs. This is perhaps not surprising since positive reframing coping is typically considered an indirect or emotional-based coping mechanism, and thus likely to correlate with other individual traits or self-perceptions. For example, research has supported that those with higher self-esteem are more likely to score higher on affective state scales (with positive reframing being an example of an affective state) than motivational states (Chen et al., 2004). Indeed, those who reported higher self-esteem and confidence in science could provide someone with the necessary internal resources to frame the pandemic in a positive light.

Finally, I examined predictors of religious coping (see Fig. 7.4).

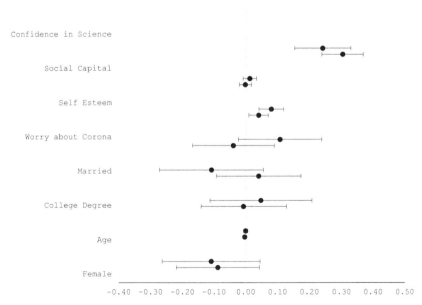

Fig. 7.3. Factors That Affect Positive Reframing Coping: The United States and Finland. *Note*: US confidence intervals are presented as the top line in chart. US RSQ = 0.118, Finnish RSQ = 0.127.

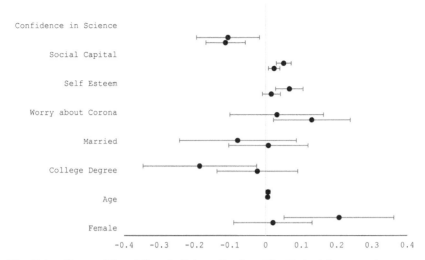

Fig. 7.4. Factors That Affect Religious Coping: The United States and Finland. *Note*: US confidence intervals are presented as the top line in chart. US RSQ = 0.108, Finnish RSQ = 0.060.

When examining the Finnish and US samples together for religious coping, the country difference was the strongest predictor, with US residents reporting the use of religious coping more than their Finnish counterparts. These findings support recent research from the Pew Research Center (2018) that US residents (and in particular US Christians) are far more likely to report that religion is important in their lives compared to Finnish residents, with 68% reporting this importance compared to 12% reporting, respectively. Given these stark differences, it is perhaps not surprising that country difference proved to be the most significant predictor for religious coping.

In the United States, citizens who are older, female, with higher self-esteem, and with higher social capital were more likely to report using religious coping during COVID-19. Those US residents who were more likely to have confidence in science and a college degree were significantly less likely to use religious coping. Comparatively, several similar predictors emerged for Finnish residents, including increased likelihood of using religious coping for older persons and those with higher social capital. Also similarly, those Finnish residents who reported higher confidence in science were less likely to use religious coping. Probably the most interesting difference is that worry about coronavirus was a significant positive predictor for Finnish residents but not for the United States. For Finnish residents, being worried about the pandemic prompted a religious approach. Comparatively, perhaps given the pervasiveness of the importance of religion in the United States, many people turned to religious coping (although remarkably less for those with college degrees or confidence in science) regardless of worry.

Table 7.1 summarizes the findings from the four analyses. During the pandemic, US citizens reported higher use of maladaptive coping and less use of

# 116   Donna Sedgwick

Table 7.1.   Summary of the Significant Predictors with Their Direction for Coping Strategies: Finland and the United States.

| | Maladaptive | | Active/Expressive and Planning | | Positive Reframing | | Religious | |
|---|---|---|---|---|---|---|---|---|
| | FIN | US | FIN | US | FIN | US | FIN | US |
| Country Difference | + | | | | – | | – | + |
| Self-esteem | – | – | | | + | + | | + |
| Confidence in Science | – | – | | | + | + | – | – |
| Female | – | – | + | + | | | | + |
| Social capital | – | | + | + | | | + | + |
| Worry about COVID-19 | | | + | + | | | + | |
| Age | – | – | – | – | | | + | + |
| College degree | | | + | + | | | | – |
| Married | | | | | | | | |

the adaptive coping strategies compared to their Finnish counterparts. Also, as expected, I found significant country difference in terms of religious coping, with US citizens reporting higher usage. Several predictors primarily correlated to beneficial outcomes – meaning they reduced the likelihood of using maladaptive coping and/or increased the use of at least one of the adaptive coping strategies. These predictors included increased self-esteem, confidence in science, being female, and worrying about COVID-19. However, these predictors varied by coping strategy and country. Additionally, I found some unexpected predictor differences by country, notably that social capital was almost a positive predictor for US residents for maladaptive coping (compared to a negative predictor for Finnish residents), and that worry about COVID-19 is a positive predictor for religious coping for Finnish residents, but not US residents.

Some interesting trends are apparent, and useful for public and mental health professions. First, while the pandemic was a unique traumatic event, those who were more worried about it did not use maladaptive coping any differently than those who did not report being as worried about the pandemic. This can allay fears that extreme worry about a pandemic may lead to negative coping strategies. Additionally, despite some prior research suggesting otherwise, our findings suggest that confidence in science acted as a protective factor that reduced the use of maladaptive coping. Thus, having health officials create clear, effective messaging early on about the science of the pandemic could help reduce negative coping mechanisms. These clear messages could also help boost positive reframing coping as confidence in science was shown to directly affect this strategy. As some studies have found a connection between self-esteem and crisis self-efficacy

(Baguri et al., 2022), creating messages that also explain what steps people can take during a pandemic to reduce their risk could also result in them creating positive reframing tactics.

However, equally important is understanding that different predictors explain variation in the two different positive coping strategies. For more active, expressive, and planning coping, confidence in science and self-esteem were not important predictors, but having higher social capital, a college degree, being female, and worrying about the pandemic did. Interestingly, worrying about the pandemic is not related to maladaptive coping, and more importantly, can lead to a positive coping strategy. Future research could investigate overall family coping approaches and if having people made up of these different individual predictors leads to a family with better coping management than others.

## Relationship Between Coping Strategies and Quality of Life

After examining predictors of the various types of coping strategies, I now turn to understanding if and how these various coping strategies affected quality of life factors. Prior research findings are mixed on whether adaptive and religious coping (direct or indirect) have a positive effect on well-being. Conversely, maladaptive coping is more consistently found to have a negative effect on well-being measures and a positive effect on stress, anxiety, and depression.

The results of some studies support that adaptive coping has positive effects on well-being and life satisfaction, including a 2022 systematic review of psychological dimensions during COVID-19 (Filindassi et al., 2022). Similarly, Budimir et al. (2021) find that positive thinking, active stress coping, and social support are positively associated with life satisfaction and negatively associated with perceived stress and anxiety. Shamblaw et al. (2021) also find that active coping and positive reframing result in lower depression and higher quality of life scores for respondents. Strongylaki et al. (2021) also find lower stress scores for respondents that report using active, positive reframing, acceptance, and use of emotional support coping strategies, and Gurvich et al. (2021) find a similar effect of positive emotion coping to decrease stress, anxiety, and depression. Finally, Wang et al. (2020) find that that positive coping styles are likely to decrease psychological distress.

However, other studies find that adaptive coping strategies have no effect on well-being outcomes or a reduced effect compared to maladaptive strategies. For example, Agha (2021) finds that both problem-focused and positive coping are insignificant predictors of well-being. Similarly, while Kirby et al. (2022) find that problem-focused coping increases well-being, it is not as consistent or as strong of a predictor in the 13 countries studied as maladaptive coping was in predicting reduced well-being.

How religious coping affects overall life quality has also resulted in mixed findings. Some studies have found a positive relationship between religious coping and negative mental health outcomes, including that religious coping can result in increased stress, anxiety, and depression (Agha, 2021; Strongylaki et al., 2021). However, while not as many studies find positive outcomes for religious coping,

## 118    Donna Sedgwick

Shamblaw et al. (2021) do find a positive relationship between religious coping and quality of life. While the literature is mixed on whether adaptive and religious coping strategies have a positive effect on well-being and quality of life, studies have found that maladaptive strategies, particularly substance use, consistently result in decreased well-being and lowered quality of life for the people that use them. For example, Wang et al. (2020) find that those people who use negative coping styles are more likely to report psychological distress. Similarly, several studies find that self-distraction, behavioral disengagement, or avoidance coping strategies, which often includes substance use as a dimension, result in decreased well-being and increased mental health issues (Agha, 2021; Gurvich et al., 2021; Kirby et al., 2022; Shamblaw et al., 2021). Some researchers specifically examine the effects of substance use coping strategies by themself and find that that people who use substances for coping report increased stress (Strongylaki et al., 2021) and depression (Shamblaw et al., 2021). Additionally, Rogowska et al. (2021) find that students who are more likely to report using negative emotional coping strategies are more likely to report lower life satisfaction. Whether active or emotional-based, maladaptive coping mechanisms negatively affect a person's overall well-being.

### Anticipated Findings

Thus, based upon the literature reviewed, I expect that those people that report using maladaptive coping strategies to report lower life satisfaction. And while not as clear if the other coping strategies will have a significant effect, I expect direct and indirect adaptive coping (expressive/active and planning and positive reframing) to have a positive effect on life satisfaction and religion coping to have a negative effect.

First, I examined predictors of quality of life before adding in the four coping strategies. I used life satisfaction at T2 (November 2020) as a proxy measure of well-being (see Kirby et al., 2022), and use predictor variables at T1, including life satisfaction at T1, to examine which factors contribute to a change in life satisfaction during that period.

Unlike the analyses run on the entire sample when examining predictors of coping strategies, country is not a significant predictor of the change in life satisfaction from April 2020 to November 2020. While there is no significant difference in change to life satisfaction between US and Finnish citizens during that time, the regression analyses separated by country revealed some different predictor variables for each country. The three main differences by country included the effects of age, being female, and worrying about the coronavirus. Female Finnish residents reported a positive change in life satisfaction during the period compared to their male counterparts, while in the United States there was no significant difference by gender. Conversely, older US residents reported a positive change in life satisfaction compared to younger residents, while having a null effect in Finland. While those differences are interesting and may speak to cultural differences, probably the most interesting difference was that worry about the coronavirus explained a decrease in life satisfaction from April 2020 to November 2020 for US residents, but not for Finnish residents. Some possible explanations for this finding include the explosion of pandemic cases in the United States compared to Finland during this time frame. Cases reached over 2 million during the summer of 2020 in the United States (CNN Editorial Research, 2024), and the United States' death rate per capita was almost twice that of Finland, reporting 344 cases per 100,000 compared to 161 cases per 100,00, respectively (Johns Hopkins, 2023).

Of course, some similarities exist also, and to no surprise, the strongest predictor in life satisfaction for both countries in November 2020 was a person's reported life satisfaction in April 2020. While the effects vary in strength, in both countries those people who were married, those who had higher self-esteem, and those who reported higher social capital and confidence in science also reported an increase in life satisfaction between April 2020 and November 2020.

Next, I included the four coping strategies to the model to see what, if any, effect that they had on change in life satisfaction from April 2020 to November 2020 (see Fig. 7.5).

When examining the regression analysis of change in life satisfaction from April 2020 to November 2020, many of the control variables continued to be significant even when including the coping strategies for both countries. Life satisfaction in April continued to be the strongest predictor in both countries. Additionally, those Finnish and US residents who were married, had higher self-esteem, or reported higher social capital were more likely to report an increase in life satisfaction from April 2020 to November 2020. Also, a couple of the differences between the countries remained in this model, with US residents

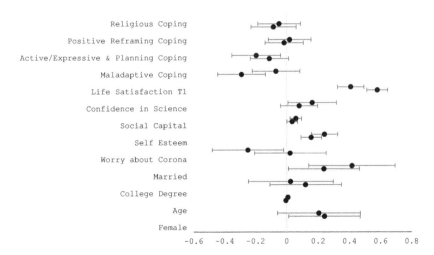

Fig. 7.5. Predictors of Change in Life Satisfaction in November 2020: The United States and Finland. *Note*: US confidence intervals are presented as the top line for each predictor. US RSQ = 0.516, Finnish RSQ = 0.567.

## 120    *Donna Sedgwick*

who reported worrying about coronavirus reporting decreased life satisfaction and Finnish females reporting an increase in life satisfaction. A new difference emerged in the model, with those with higher confidence in science reporting an increase in life satisfaction for US residents but not for Finnish residents. Additionally, age as a predictor was no longer a significant predictor for change in life satisfaction in either country.

Regarding the effect of the coping strategies on life satisfaction, I found mixed results from what I expected. As expected, those who reported using maladaptive strategies in April 2020 showed a significant decrease in life satisfaction in November 2020; however, this finding was only significant for Finnish residents. These results are consistent with a multitude of prior studies (Agha, 2021; Gurvich et al., 2021; Kirby et al., 2022; Shamblaw et al., 2021). That maladaptive strategies did not decrease life satisfaction for US residents was an unexpected finding. As discussed above, it could be that with the overall increase in alcohol use for US residents during this timeframe, it lessened the typical impact that this type of coping had on life satisfaction. In other words, it could be that this type of coping was used as more of a social outlet in a time when social outlets were minimal, and thus reduced the overall negative effect. Or perhaps increased alcohol usage overall reduced the stigma of admitting to using alcohol as a way "to deal" with the pandemic, which in turn reduced its typical correlation to reduced life satisfaction. This finding warrants further investigation.

Additionally, while not completely unexpected, since as discussed above adaptive coping does not always produce positive effects on quality-of-life variables, I was surprised to find that Finnish (trending toward significance at $p = 0.08$) and US residents ($p < 0.05$) who reported using Active/Expressive and Planning coping also reported a decrease in life satisfaction from April 2020 to November 2020. This coping strategy includes tactics such as seeking advice or comfort from friends and family and turning to work or developing plans in response to the pandemic. However, it also includes expressing negative thoughts and feelings. While I anticipated that the adaptive coping could have a null effect (and indeed, this is what I found for positive reframing), I did not expect this positive direct coping strategy to have a significant negative effect. These findings could mirror those found by Rogowska et al. (2021) that emotion-oriented coping (which in the coping scale they used included negative emotional responses) can result in decreased life satisfaction. However, our active/expressive and planning measure also includes other coping mechanisms besides the negative expression of emotions. Another possible explanation is that those people who participated in these direct coping strategies in April 2020 found themselves still dealing with the realities of a pandemic in November 2020. In other words, despite their direct attempts, their "planning" did not alter their current reality and/or their "negative feelings" persisted (as did the pandemic). Also, while they may have sought comfort from family or friends, the social distancing in place could have limited the ease with which this method could be enacted (Agha, 2021; Clair et al., 2021). In other words, it could be that the longevity and physical reality of the pandemic rendered this coping strategy as less effective, and ultimately resulted in decreased life satisfaction.

## Conclusion

Relying on TTSC framework, this chapter analyzed individual coping in two nations during the first year of COVID-19 pandemic. Generally, the findings of our comparative study on the predictors of various coping mechanisms and their effects on the change in life satisfaction during the pandemic's first year raise questions for future research. The context of the pandemic may have created a unique situation that rendered coping mechanisms to behave in unusual ways. For public health and mental health professionals, this means that caution may be warranted in promoting the typical direct-action adaptive approaches as a safeguard for most individuals. Also, it might suggest that public health officials encourage friends and family members to heed seriously when others reach out to them for support or share their negative feelings about the pandemic. These expressions and actions could be more than just "blowing off steam," and point to the need for active support (which can be challenging during the social distancing mandated during the pandemic).

Additionally, even when controlling for a multitude of coping mechanisms, several personal resources proved important for an increase in life satisfaction and can be promoted as valuable means to safeguard against the negative social consequences of a pandemic. When people feel a strong sense of social capital, their life satisfaction increases. Encouraging creative ways to still build a sense of community during a pandemic can improve people's lives. Also, typical mental health indicators, such as self-esteem, should continue to be monitored during the pandemic, for those that had increased self-esteem appeared to navigate the early months of the pandemic better.

## References

Agha, S. (2021). Mental well-being and association of the four factors coping structure model: A perspective of people living in lockdown during COVID-19. *Ethics, Medicine and Public Health, 16*, 100605, 1–8.

Alaszewski, A. (2023). *Managing risk during the COVID-19 pandemic: Global policies, narratives and practices*. Bristol University Press.

Baguri, E. M., Roslan, S., Hassan, S. A., Krauss, S. E., & Zaremohzzabieh, Z. (2022). How do self-esteem, dispositional hope, crisis self-efficacy, mattering, and gender differences affect teacher resilience during COVID-19 school closures?. *International Journal of Environmental Research and Public Health, 19*(7), 4150.

Budimir, S., Probst, T., & Pieh, C. (2021). Coping strategies and mental health during COVID-19 lockdown. *Journal of Mental Health, 30*(2), 156–163.

Carver, C. S. (1997). You want to measure coping but your protocol' too long: Consider the brief cope. *International Journal of Behavioral Medicine, 4*(1), 92–100.

Chen, C., Guan, Z., Sun, L., Zhou, T., & Guan, R. (2022). COVID-19 exposure, pandemic-related appraisals, coping strategies, and psychological symptoms among the frontline medical staff and gender differences in coping processes. *Applied Cognitive Psychology, 36*(1), 111–120.

Chen, G., Stanley, M. G., & Eden, D. (2004). General self-efficacy and self-esteem: toward theoretical and empirical distinction between correlated self-evaluations. *Journal of Organizational Behavior, 25*(3), 375–395.

## 122 Donna Sedgwick

Clair, R., Gordon, M., Kroon, M., & Reilly, C. (2021). The effects of social isolation on well-being and life satisfaction during pandemic. *Humanities and Social Sciences Communications*, 8(1), 1–6.

CNN Editorial Research. (2024, January 2). *Covid-19 pandemic timeline fast facts.* https://www.cnn.com/2021/08/09/health/covid-19-pandemic-timeline-fast-facts/index.html

Coiro, M. J., Watson, K. H., Ciriegio, A., Jones, M., Wolfson, A. R., Reisman, J., & Compas, B. E. (2021). Coping with COVID-19 stress: Associations with depression and anxiety in a diverse sample of U.S. adults. *Current Psychology*, 42, 11497–11509.

David, A., Park, C. L., Awao, S., Vega, S., Zuckerman, M., White, T., & Hanna, D. (2022). Religiousness in the first year of COVID-19: A systematic review of empirical research. *Current Research in Ecological and Social Psychology*, 100075.

Denisse, M. M., Bertha, M. R. R., Oscar, M. P., & Nataly, F. R. (2020). Coping responses During the COVID-19 pandemic: A cross-cultural comparison of Russia, Kyrgyzstan, and Peru. *Psychology in Russia: State of the Art*, 13(4), 55–74.

Fallahi, C. R., Blau, J. J. C., Mitchell, M. T., Rodrigues, H. A., Daigle, C. D., Heinze, A. M., LaChance, A., & DeLeo, L. (2021). Understanding the pandemic experience for people with a preexisting mental health disorder. *Traumatology*, 27(4), 471–478.

Filindassi, V., Pedrini, C., Sabadini, C., Duradoni, M., & Guazzini, A. (2022). Impact of COVID-19 first wave on psychological and psychosocial dimensions: A systematic review. *Covid*, 2(3), 273–340.

Fluharty, M., & Fancourt, D (2021). How have people been coping during the COVID-19 pandemic? Patterns and predictors of coping strategies amongst 26,016 UK adults. *BMC Psychology*, 9(107), 1–12.

Gurvich, C., Thomas, N., Thomas, E. H., Hudaib, A. R., Sood, L., Fabiatos, K., Sutton, K., Isaacs, A., Arunogiri, S., Sharp, G., & Kulkarni, J. (2021). Coping styles and mental health in response to societal changes during the COVID-19 pandemic. *International Journal of Social Psychiatry*, 67(5), 540–549.

Horesh, D., & Brown, A. D. (2020). Traumatic stress in the age of COVID-19: A call to close critical gaps and adapt to new realities. *Psychological Trauma: Theory, Research, Practice, and Policy*, 12(4), 331–335.

Huy, N. T., Nguyen Tran, M. D., Mohammed Alhady, S. T., Luu, M. N., Hassan, A. K., Giang, T. V., Truong, L. V., Ravikulan, R., Raut, A. P., Dayyab, F. M., Durme, S. P., Trang, V. T., Loc, L. Q., & Thach, P. N. (2021). Perceived stress of quarantine and isolation during COVID-19 pandemic: A global survey. *Frontiers in Psychiatry*, 12, 651.

Javed, S., & Parveen, H. (2021). Adaptive coping strategies used by people during coronavirus. *Journal of Education and Health Promotion*, 10, 1–8.

Jean-Baptiste, C. O., Herring, R. P., Beeson, W. L., Dos Santos, H., & Banta, J. E. (2020). Stressful life events and social capital during the early phase of COVID-19 in the US. *Social Sciences & Humanities Open*, 2(1), 100057, 1–10.

John Hopkins University & Medicine. (2023, March 10). *Mortality analysis.* https://coronavirus.jhu.edu/data/mortality

Kirby, L. D., Qian, W., Adiguzel, Z., Afshar Jahanshahi, A., Bakracheva, M., Orejarena Ballestas, M. C., Cruz, J. F. A., Dash, A., Dias, C., Ferreira, M. J., Goosen, J. G., Kamble, S. V., Mihaylov, N. L., Pan, F., Sofia, R., Stallen, M., Tamir, M., van Dijk, W. W., Vitterso, J., & Smith, C. A. (2022). Appraisal and coping predict health and well-being during the COVID-19 pandemic: An international approach. *International Journal of Psychology*, 57(1), 49–62.

Krase, K., Luzuriaga, L., Wang, D., Schoolnik, A., Parris-Strigle, C., Attis, L., & Brown, P. (2022). Exploring the impact of gender on challenges and coping during the COVID-19 pandemic. *International Journal of Sociology and Social Policy*, 42(11–12), 1001–1012.

## Coping, Well-being, and COVID-19   123

Lazarus, R. S., & Folkman, S. (1984). *Stress, appraisal, and coping.* Springer publishing company.

Lee, B. P., Dodge, J. L., Leventhal, A., & Terrault, N. A. (2021). Retail alcohol and tobacco sales during COVID-19. *Annals of Internal Medicine, 174*(7), 1027–1029.

Lueger-Schuster, B., Zrnić Novaković, I., & Lotzin, A. (2022). Two years of COVID-19 in Austria—Exploratory longitudinal study of mental health outcomes and coping behaviors in the general population. *International Journal of Environmental Research and Public Health, 19*(13), 8223, 1–18.

Maestripieri, L. (2021). The Covid-19 pandemics: Why intersectionality matters. *Frontiers in Sociology, 6*(642662), 1–6.

Meyer, D., Van Rheenen, T. E., Neill, E., Phillipou, A., Tan, E. J., Toh, W. L., ... & Rossell, S. L. (2022). Surviving the COVID-19 pandemic: An examination of adaptive coping strategies. *Heliyon, 8*(5), e09508.

Mohamed, N. H., Beckstein, A., Tze Ping Pang, N., Hutchings, P. B., Dawood, S. R. S., Fadilah, R., Sullivan, K., Yahaya, A., & Baral, J. E. V. (2022). Cross-cultural differences in psychological health, perceived stress, and coping strategies of university students during the COVID-19 pandemic. *European Journal of Mental Health, 17*(2), 65–77.

Munsell, S. E., O'Malley, L., & Mackey, C. (2020). Coping with COVID. *Educational Research: Theory and Practice, 31*(3), 101–109.

Partouche-Sebban, J., Rezaee Vessal, S., Sorio, R., Castellano, S., Khelladi, I., & Orhan, M. A. (2021). How death anxiety influences coping strategies during the COVID-19 pandemic: investigating the role of spirituality, national identity, lockdown and trust. *Journal of Marketing Management, 37*(17–18), 1815–1839.

Peacock, E. J., & Wong, P.T.P. (1990). The stress appraisal measure (SAM): a multidimensional approach to cognitive appraisal. *Stress Medicine, 6*, 227–236.

Pew Research Center. (2018). The age gap in religion around the world. (June 13, 2018). https://www.pewresearch.org/religion/2018/06/13/the-age-gap-in-religion-around-the-world/.

Rogowska, A. M., Kuśnierz, C., & Ochnik, D. (2021). Changes in stress, coping styles, and life satisfaction between the first and second waves of the COVID-19 pandemic: A longitudinal cross-lagged study in a sample of university students. *Journal of Clinical Medicine, 10*(17), 4025, 1–22.

Schillinger, A. M., & Stalpers, C. (2021). Mediation effect of adaptive coping between self-esteem and loneliness in college students. Unpublished Manuscript. Tilburg University.

Seid, A. K., Hesse, M., & Bloomfield, K. (2016). 'Make it another for me and my mates': Does social capital encourage risky drinking among the Danish general population?. *Scandinavian Journal of Public Health, 44*(3), 240–248.

Shamblaw, A. L., Rumas, R. L., & Best, M. W. (2021). Coping during the COVID-19 pandemic: Relations with mental health and quality of life. *Canadian Psychology/Psychologie Canadienne, 62*(1), 92–100.

Snel, E., Engbersen, G., de Boom, J., & van Bochove, M. (2022). Social capital as protection against the mental health impact of the COVID-19 pandemic. *Frontiers in Sociology, 7*, 728541.

Solberg, M. A., Gridley, M. K., & Peters, R. M. (2022). The factor structure of the brief cope: A systematic review. *Western Journal of Nursing Research, 44*(6), 612–627.

Strongylaki, N. P., Pilafas, G., Dermati, A., Menti, D., & Lyrakos, G. (2021). Effect of coping strategies on acute stress during the COVID-19 pandemic in Greece. *Health & Research Journal, 7*(3), 98–108.

Vos, J. (2021). *The psychology of COVID-19: Building resilience for future pandemics* (1st ed.). SAGE.

## 124    Donna Sedgwick

Wang, H., Xia, Q., Xiong, Z., Li, Z., Xiang, W., Yuan, Y., Liu, Y., & Li, Z. (2020) The psychological distress and coping styles in the early stages of the 2019 coronavirus disease (COVID-19) epidemic in the general mainland Chinese population: A web-based survey. *PLoS ONE, 15*(5), e0233410.

World Health Organization. (2022, March 2). *Mental health and Covid-19. Early evidence of the pandemic's impact.* https://www.who.int/publications/i/item/WHO-2019-nCoV-Sci_Brief-Mental_health-2022

Wilczyńska, A., Januszek, M., & Bargiel-Matusiewicz, K. (2015). The need of belonging and sense of belonging versus effectiveness of coping. *Polish Psychological Bulletin, 46*(1), 72–81.

Chapter 8

# Compliance with Protective Health Behaviors During COVID-19: Variations Over Time and by Country

*Donna Sedgwick*

*Virginia Tech, USA*

### Abstract

This chapter documents how the early request for citizens to participate in health-protective behaviors to quell the spread of the disease became politicized. Health-protective behaviors, such as social distancing and mask wearing, were found to reduce the spread of COVID-19. Yet, despite the evidence that compliance helped control the pandemic's spread, mask wearing became a politicized symbol during the early stages of the pandemic. Particularly in the United States, bipartisan stances for and against mask wearing developed quickly as conspiracy theories, supported by President Trump, downplayed the seriousness of the pandemic. As vaccines appeared by late 2020, this polarization continued, again with President Trump aiming blame that the release of the vaccine was timed with 2020 election and raising questions with its safety. In comparison, Prime Minister Marin took a pro-science, global approach to Finland's mandate and vaccine response. Using regression analysis, I examine the growing political divide that occurred between April 2020 and November 2020, highlighting the growth of politicization for both mask wearing and vaccine intention in both the United States and Finland. While analyses from April 2020 show support for the party in power (Republicans for the United States and left-leaning parties for Finland) was not a significant predictor of mask wearing in either country, by November 2020, political party significantly predicted both mask wearing and vaccine intention in

---

Perceptions of a Pandemic: A Cross-Continental Comparison of Citizen Perceptions, Attitudes, and Behaviors During COVID-19, 125–141
Copyright © 2025 by Donna Sedgwick
Published under exclusive licence by Emerald Publishing Limited
doi:10.1108/978-1-83608-624-620241008

## 126    *Donna Sedgwick*

both countries. Additionally, other important predictive factors, particularly state/citizen collaborative dimensions, are reviewed and discussed.

*Keywords*: Health-protective behaviors; collaboration theory; compliance; trust in institutions; symbolic interaction theory

## Introduction

In the early response to the pandemic, citizens were asked to participate in health-protective behaviors to quell the spread of the disease. Indeed, health-protective behaviors, such as social distancing and mask wearing, were found to reduce the spread of COVID-19 (Brooks & Butler, 2021; Delen et al., 2020). Many researchers found that typical attitudinal factors, such as worry about becoming ill, trust in institutions, and social capital, affected the likelihood of compliance (Hao et al., 2021). Scholars also discovered that exposure to multiple media news outlets (social media, print, or broadcast news) and selection of media type (mainstream vs conservative) affected willingness to comply with health-protective behaviors (Koivula et al., 2023). How requests and mandates were written to inspire the public to comply with health-protective behaviors also mattered (Bolsen & Palm, 2022; Lin et al., 2020). Additionally, factors such as collaborative dimensions in the state–citizen relationship also played a significant role (Sedgwick et al., 2022).

Ultimately, while non-medicinal health preventative measures played an important part in public health management of the disease, the development of vaccines was a vital step in bringing the pandemic to an end. Indeed, as Albrecht (2022, p. 2) observed, "vaccines have saved more lives than any other medical technology." However, during the first year of the pandemic, scholars observed a declining rate of receptivity for the vaccine, with higher reported uptake agreement in April 2020 than in October 2020 (Lin et al., 2020). Many factors may explain this change of heart for the public, but a primary factor was the politicization of the pandemic itself. This politization included questioning its origin and severity at first, but then extended to questioning the efficacy of the containment measures, particularly mask wearing, social distancing, and eventually, the vaccine.

In this chapter, I discuss the importance of health-protective behaviors, including vaccines, and the typical explanations that predict compliance. However, I explore the unique situation that arose with COVID-19: the politization of the disease and its preventative measures. I examine the change in the importance of political party as a predictive factor in a short amount of time (from April 2020 until November 2020). I suggest that through a variety of interactions, such as citizens observing world leaders like former President Donald Trump downplaying the severity of the pandemic and engaging with conspiracy theories on various media outlets about the efficacy of health-protective behaviors, masks and vaccines became strong symbols that came to represent one's political ideology and relationship between themselves and the State. Thus, I ask, how did mask

# Compliance with Protective Health Behaviors    *127*

wearing compliance change over time, and what factors explain compliance in Finland and the United States? Second, I ask what factors shaped intended vaccine uptake for both nations?

## The Importance of Health-Protective Behaviors and Compliance

Like past global pandemics, public health officials called for the public to engage with health-protective behaviors to stop the spread of COVID-19. Health-protective behaviors, such as hand washing, mask wearing, and social distancing, were also recommended for prior outbreaks, such as SARS, H1N1, and Swine Flu (Burgess & Horii, 2012; Cava et al., 2005; Prati et al., 2011; Rubin et al., 2009; St-Amant et al., 2021). These protective behaviors reduce disease spread by minimizing contact with others, decreasing the input and output spread of droplets, or increasing the likelihood of killing the virus before spread can occur. These behaviors are often viewed as stop gap measures until vaccines and treatment drugs are readily available for the public (Lin et al., 2020); however, mask wearing, in particular, provides a proactive measure to prevent disease spread while attempting to resume pre-pandemic public life (St-Amant et al., 2021). During the COVID-19 pandemic, some of these health protocols turned into mandates, with city-wide issued curfews and lockdowns (Morrison, 2020), social distancing implemented once re-opening occurred (Pearce, 2020), and requirements for mask wearing when in public spaces (Jacobs & Ohinmaa, 2020). Indeed, findings suggest a reduction in COVID-19 cases connected to social distancing and mask wearing (Brooks & Butler, 2021; Delen et al., 2020).

The request for citizens to wear masks varied by country, aligning with the rate of infection and spread in that country. Subsequently, scholars identified differences in uptake rates of mask usage cross-nationally (St-Amant et al., 2021). Given its importance in disease reduction during the early phases of the pandemic, I analyze self-reported mask-wearing at two points, April 2020 and November 2020, for a panel samples in Finland and the United States. The question used was a four-point Likert scale asking about wearing a mask in public, with a score of 4 indicating strongest compliance. I also conducted a paired samples *t*-test to examine if the mean difference in compliance changed over that period. See Table 8.1 for the mean compliance and difference with mask wearing in Finland and the United States in April 2020 and November 2020.

Table 8.1.   Mean Compliance and Difference with Mask Wearing in Finland and the United States, April 2020 and November 2020.

|  | April 2020 | November 2020 | Mean Difference |
|---|---|---|---|
| Finland (*n* = 767) | 1.49 | 2.81 | 1.32*** |
| The United States (*n* = 609) | 3.05 | 3.53 | 0.478*** |

## 128   Donna Sedgwick

Examining the average face mask wearing shows a statistically significant increase for both Finland and the United States, although the rate of compliance increases more for Finnish citizens. This increase for Finland is most likely due to relatively minimal infection rate early in the pandemic for Finland, which led to decreased uptake of mask wearing compared to the United States. Additionally, unlike Asian cultures, such as China, Japan, and Taiwan, where mask wearing is considered a typical action taken by citizens in the prevention of most illnesses (Burgess & Horii, 2012; St-Amant et al., 2021), mask wearing is not a culturally embedded process in response to public health safety in Finland and the United States. Indeed, some scholars identify a Western anti-mask stance connected to racist anti-Asian sentiments that came about with the onset of the pandemic (Ren & Feagin, 2021).

Despite the underlying stance toward mask wearing, the request for citizens to wear a mask publicly in the United States and Finland was a new request (at least since the Spanish Flu pandemic of 1918; French, 2020). While the rate of increase in mask wearing for the United States is not as high, this is perhaps explained simply by the higher compliance earlier in the pandemic but could also possibly be explained by declining support for health-protective behaviors during the April 2020–November 2020 period (Barry et al., 2021). Given the importance of health-protective behaviors to quell the spread of disease, I briefly turn to an overview of factors that affect compliance. Additionally, I draw attention to a symbolic-interactionist framework to explore how the pandemic, mask wearing, and vaccines became salient symbols of political ideology, which in turn changed the importance of political party as a predictive factor in compliance in the initial stages of the pandemic.

## Typical Factors that Affect Compliance with Health-Protective Behaviors

Scholars frequently study factors that affect compliance to health-protective behaviors as those behaviors slow the spread of disease. While many examinations consider a multitude of factors, predictive factors typically fall into three broad categories: trust in institutions, such as government and science; peer pressures and social capital; and rational choice behaviors (Sedgwick et al., 2022). When citizens trust in institutions, such as governments and science, they deem the demands made by the state as legitimate and are generally more willing to comply (Braithwaite & Makkai, 1994; Im et al., 2014; Marien & Hooghe, 2011). Indeed, prior studies typically support that when citizens trust in institutions their compliance to health-protective protocols increases (Bish & Michie, 2010; Rubin et al., 2009; Tang & Wong, 2003), although some mixed results also exist (Chuang et al., 2015; Prati et al., 2011; Travaglino & Moon, 2021).

Social pressures to conform to mandates requested by governments also act as powerful forces to bring about compliance to health-protective behaviors (Bish & Michie, 2010; van Rooij et al., 2020). Two important processes shape how these social norms work. Citizens either observe or perceive that others are complying, or they internalize what they believe others expect of them. If citizens' tight-knit

Compliance with Protective Health Behaviors   *129*

social networks include a pro-normative stance toward compliance, then they too are more likely to comply. Indeed, bonding social capital is a consistent positive predictor for compliance to health-protective behaviors (Chuang et al., 2015).

However, attitudes toward institutions and pressures from social networks are not the only factors that matter. Studies consistently find that worry about the severity of the illness, citizens' ability to comply with the requested mandates, and fears of fines also shape compliance outcomes (Bish & Michie, 2010; Chuang et al., 2015; Prati et al., 2011; Quinn et al., 2009; Rubin et al., 2009). In other words, rational choice factors also shape if and how people comply; although, perhaps what was not expected in the COVID-19 pandemic was how seemingly objective concerns about the severity of the pandemic would be shaped by citizens' trust in institutions and their self-selected social networks (Koskan et al., 2023). To that end, "worrying about the illness," or even belief in the existence of the pandemic overall, became less about a rational assessment of disease and more about how belief in that disease became a symbol that reflected one's belief in science and government compared to others who downplayed its severity and saw it as a symbol of conspiracy that infringed upon personal freedoms (St-Amant et al., 2021).

## Symbolic Interactionism and the COVID-19 Pandemic

The symbolic interactionist approach offers an understanding of how society operates that is rooted at the micro-level. Theorists such as George Mead (1934) and Howard Blumer (1969) contend that society is continually constructed through ongoing relationship interactions, during which shared language, norms, and symbols develop to guide an understanding of those interactions and the surrounding situations. Blumer (1969) focuses on how meanings are not inherent in objects, but develop, and potentially change, through ongoing interactions.

Sedgwick et al. (2022) build on a symbolic interactionist approach in their study of compliance to health-protective behaviors by arguing that collaborative dimensions that underscore an envisioned relationship between citizens and the state offer predictive insight to compliance with COVID-19 health-protective behaviors. In fact, their findings support that for both the United States and Finland, citizens who report that they and others have a role in concert with the state to combat the pandemic are more likely to comply with social distancing and hand washing protocols. In other words, when citizens envision interactions with the state that include their responsibility in combatting the pandemic, they report more compliance, even when controlling for typical social capital, trust in institutions, and rational choice factors. Another noteworthy point is that for both countries, political party is not a predictive variable for compliance (Sedgwick et al., 2022). I highlight this finding for the United States because this null finding indicates that citizens who were aligned with the political party of then President Trump (Republicans) and citizens who were members of the political party in opposition (Democrats) could both imagine the state as a meaningful entity, larger than the presidency alone. Factors other than political party, including this understanding of a collaborative role for citizens in combatting the pandemic, also matter for understanding compliance.

## 130  *Donna Sedgwick*

However, the Sedgwick and associate research was conducted very early in the pandemic (April 2020) and only looked at social distancing and hand washing behaviors (due to mask wearing in Finland being very minimal during this time). Many scholars document a changing tide that occurred during the pandemic, as a growing number of citizens, particularly those in the United States who aligned themselves with President Trump's dismissiveness of the seriousness of the pandemic, became less likely to comply with health-protective behaviors (Barry et al., 2021; Bierwiaczonek et al., 2020; Nocera & McLean, 2023). Scholars focused on other European countries also note these shifting beliefs about the responses to the pandemic (Bernacer et al., 2021).

Given these trends of shifting sentiments, I turn my attention to an analysis to compare factors that affected mask wearing for both US and Finish citizens at two points in time, in April 2020 and November 2020. I ask how these factors change in importance as predictors. To do so, I conduct linear regression analyses on panel samples of US and Finish citizens for both timeframes. Table 8.2 reports the standardized betas and significance levels for both points in time.

Table 8.2 reveals some important similarities and changes that occurred between April 2020 and November 2020 regarding citizen compliance with mask wearing. Regarding similarities, worry about COVID-19 remained a significant positive predictor for mask wearing in both countries at both points in time. In fact, it is the only consistent predictor and lends support to others' findings that worry about an illness often promotes compliance with health-protective behaviors (Lin et al., 2020). Interestingly, while social capital has often been found to promote compliance, it was only a significant positive predictor in April 2020, and it was significant only for Finnish residents. Citizens' confidence in science was also an interesting finding because it is an inconsistent predictor. For Americans, it was not significant in April 2020, but it was a significant positive predictor in November 2020. For Finnish citizens, it was a negative predictor of compliance in April 2020 but is insignificant in November 2020. While this finding for Finnish residents in April is unexpected, it could reflect that those people who are typically confident in science held off on compliance due to changing guidelines early in the pandemic about the efficacy of mask wearing (St-Amant et al., 2021).

One striking change in these findings is the rise in importance of political party as a predictive factor for compliance to mask wearing. In April 2020, citizens who reported the same political party as the president or prime minister in power (Republicans for President Trump in the United States and Social Democratic Party, Centre Party, Green League, Left Alliance, and Swedish People's Party (left-leaning parties) for Prime Minister Marin in Finland) were no more or less likely to wear a mask than those who did not support the party in power. In other words, political party was not a significant predictor of mask wearing in either country. However, this finding changes only seven months later. By November 2020, political party became a significant predictor in both countries. The effect of the factor was in opposite directions; Republicans in the United States were significantly *less likely* to wear masks compared to democrats and others, and in Finland, the left leaning parties were significantly *more likely* to wear masks compared to citizens reporting other political parties.

## Compliance with Protective Health Behaviors 131

Table 8.2. Factors That Affect Compliance with Mask Wearing April 2020 and November 2020.

| | The United States | | Finland | |
|---|---|---|---|---|
| | *April 2020* | *November 2020* | *April 2020* | *November 2020* |
| *Collaborative dimensions* | | | | |
| Understand role | 0.027 | 0.111* | –0.050 | –0.002 |
| Easily find information | 0.045 | –0.047 | –0.082* | –0.008 |
| COVID-19 guidelines easy to follow | 0.162*** | 0.046 | 0.051 | 0.032 |
| Combat if everyone follows guidelines | –0.039 | 0.126** | –0.002 | 0.002 |
| Follow to protect myself/ family | 0.132** | 0.019 | –0.009 | 0.097 |
| Follow to protect my community | 0.248*** | 0.080 | 0.189*** | 0.131* |
| Following guidelines are challenging | 0.048 | 0.000 | 0.213*** | 0.025 |
| *Other factors* | | | | |
| Support political party in power | –0.045 | –0.118** | 0.023 | 0.084* |
| Worry about COVID-19 | 0.176*** | 0.175*** | 0.097* | 0.162*** |
| Social capital | 0.012 | 0.021 | 0.154*** | 0.034 |
| Confidence in science | 0.032 | 0.175*** | –0.174*** | 0.041 |
| *Controls* | | | | |
| Female | 0.051 | 0.059 | –0.056 | 0.071* |
| Age | 0.027 | 0.016 | –0.061 | 0.029 |
| Married | –0.078** | 0.028 | –0.017 | 0.079* |
| College degree | 0.024 | 0.047 | 0.056 | 0.046 |

$*p < 0.05$; $** p < 0.01$; $*** p < 0.001$.

*Note*: All models are significant with RSQs ranging from 0.12 to 0.39.

Another important finding is that while more of the collaborative dimensions were significant predictors in April 2020, at least one dimension maintained significance in November 2020. Thus, despite the rise in importance of political party in significance, in both the United States and Finland, citizens who saw their collaborative role in relation to the state as one that calls upon the larger citizenry to combat the pandemic – either identifying that everyone coming together to follow

## 132   Donna Sedgwick

guidelines can combat the pandemic or that they themselves comply with mask wearing for their community – were more likely to comply with mask wearing.

These findings reflect an interesting dynamic and speak to how symbolic interactionism offers a framework to make sense of these similarities and changes. On one hand, citizen compliance is rooted in an ongoing perceived interaction between the citizen and the state about expected behaviors (Braithwaite & Makkai, 1994). As citizens perceive that the state trusts in them to do "what is expected," then they are more likely to do so. While not as many of the collaborative dimensions remain as significant predictors, perceived expectations about citizens' roles to contribute to a greater good and respond to demands from their governments exist and compel compliance with mask wearing.

On the other hand, I find the rise of importance in political party to predict compliance with mask wearing. St-Amant et al. (2021) discuss how the mask became a powerful symbol during the pandemic, changing from a functional object long used in the medical field to stop the spread of disease to having symbolic meaning that aligned with political ideology. To this point, they say: "Somehow this seemingly benign utilitarian object has acquired cultural symbolisms beyond its clearly functional purpose … [reflecting] misinformation, conspiracy, claims, and partisanship" (p. 101). Similarly, Clark and Bain-Selbo (2022) identify that, for some, refusal to wear a mask becomes a sign of their "righteous allegiance to their political tribe" (p. 161).

In the United States, and other countries as well, the mask transitioned from an object with a functional purpose to reflecting the political ideology of the wearer. How did this "seemingly benign" (St-Amant et al., 2021) object turn into a powerful symbol? First, in the United States, then President Trump publicly questioned the severity of the disease and the efficacy of masks to stop the spread of the coronavirus. For example, many scholars observe that Donald Trump disparaged mask wearing from the beginning of the pandemic (Albrecht, 2022; Bolsen & Palm, 2022; Romer & Jamieson, 2021), and Lupton et al. (2021) contend that Donald Trump equated mask wearing to weakness. However, it was not only that mask wearing was linked to cowardice, but Donald Trump and his administration actively called into question the science regarding COVID-19 overall, and subsequently, the approaches taken that would reduce disease spread. To that end, Bolsen and Palm (2022, p. 84) note that a subcommittee identified 47 times when the US federal government interfered with scientific advice about combatting COVID-19. While science contains inherent uncertainties that leave it open for question and improvement (Bolsen & Palm, 2022; Vos, 2021), President Trump, his administration, and many Republican politicians actively undermined science in their public speeches made about the pandemic (Albrecht, 2022; Bolsen & Palm, 2022; Romer & Jamieson, 2021). Indeed, as prior research has supported a connection between belief in science and political ideology, with Democrats having more optimism in science and Republicans having more pessimism in science (and greater belief in conspiracy theories) (Kang et al., 2023; Porteny et al., 2022), the mask became not only a symbol of a person's ideology, but also represented their willingness (or not) to believe in science.

*Compliance with Protective Health Behaviors* **133**

That a shift in public sentiment toward mask wearing occurred as prominent leaders disparaged its efficacy is not surprising, as past examples of the public responding to leaders' calls for action that are not supported by scientific evidence exist. For example, a majority of US citizens followed suit and labeled the US drug problem as the most important issue facing the nation by the late 1980s, in responses to Presidents Reagan and Bush sounding the alarm on this issue, despite falling drug usage rates in the United States (Alexander, 2012; Hawdon, 2001). The point is that the use of language by powerful leaders is persuasive and can bring about behavioral and attitudinal changes in constituents.

In the case of COVID-19 and mask wearing, supporters of President Trump responded to the ongoing messaging that COVID-19 was being exaggerated and that the science behind combatting COVID-19 was faulty. Through ongoing speeches, President Trump helped construct a new meaning given to the mask that represented intrusiveness by and subservience to the government by participating in its use (St-Amant et al., 2021). Consequently, those that opposed Trump also responded to this language, but in a different way. For this group of citizens, engaging in mask wearing also came to mean more than the simple utilitarian function to stop disease spread: the mask symbolized a belief in science and a political ideology (Democrat) that was in opposition to Trump's rhetoric and Trump himself. Findings support these differences in mask usage, as Barry et al. (2021) identify statistically significant differences between US Republicans and Democrats in their reported mask usage. These differences in meaning assigned to mask usage by political party are tied to the social construction of symbols and how people's identities intersect with interpretations and meanings that are assigned to those symbols. To this point, St-Amant et al. (2021, p. 108) argue that "meaning ascribed to a facemask becomes activated when it signals something about us to others."

While President Trump's anti-mask rhetoric is well known, he was not the only global leader to take a nationalist, anti-science approach to controlling disease within a country's borders (He & Chen, 2021). Brazilian President Bolsonaro and British Prime Minister Boris Johnson also used language, or concealed disease data, that downplayed the severity of the disease (He & Chen, 2021). Far-right General Secretary Ortega Smith (of the Spanish VOX party) discussed his "Spanish antibodies" being able to fight off the coronavirus (Richards, 2022). Responses like President Trump's and the others mentioned here reflect hyper-nationalist sentiments that prioritize national border safety and economic stability over a globalist viewpoint that prioritizes public well-being and science (He & Chen, 2021; Richards, 2022).

In contrast to President Trump and other right-leaning world leaders, Finland's Prime Minister Marin adopted more of a globalist viewpoint. For example, she relied on her experts such as the Minister of Social Affairs and Health. She also referred to the virus using its scientific name and frequently provided scientifically based health information about the virus and the pandemic (see Koljonen & Palonen, 2021; Lindholm et al., 2023). She also was far more likely to use appeals that focused on compassion and social cohesion than were leaders like President Trump (Dada et al., 2021). It is therefore predictable that Trump-supporting Americans were unlikely to wear masks while Marin-following Finns were more likely to wear masks.

## 134    Donna Sedgwick

Conservative broadcast news and social media outlets also relayed conspiracy theories about the efficacy and safety of preventative measures, which often fortified oppositional attitudes and behaviors toward them (Richards, 2022). For example, Albrecht (2022) observes that fake reports on social media, such as the vaccines affecting DNA or hurting fertility, were released concurrently with vaccine approval. Subsequently, in a study of US citizens, Romer and Jamieson (2021) find that exposure to conservative media predicted citizens' beliefs in conspiracy theories and reduced intent to uptake preventative measures. Similarly, in a comparative study of US and Finnish residents, Koivula et al. (2023) find that citizens in both countries who solely used social media as their media source, where conspiracy theories and fake news are often left unchecked (Vosoughi et al., 2018), were less likely to participate in health preventative behaviors. Conversely, those citizens who were exposed to messaging that supported the science behind COVID-19 and the related health preventative behaviors, associated mostly with mainstream broadcast news, were more likely to partake in health preventative behaviors and express vaccine intention (Adhikari et al., 2022; Latkin et al., 2023). Interestingly, Vos (2021) argues that while some attempts were made by media giants like Facebook to flag reports as "fake," this action can add more fuel to conspiracy theorists by raising suspicions by believers that the "real truth" is being censored. Thus, once conspiracy theorizing starts on social media, trying to retract those interactions and symbolic meaning making from happening can be challenging.

In short, the exchange of ideas and information from national leaders and media sources contributed to the creation of masks and vaccines as powerful symbols reflecting citizens' ideas about how political ideology, trust in science, and governmental authority interact to either compel or dissuade citizens from complying with health-protective mandates (St-Amant et al., 2021).

## Factors Affecting Vaccine Uptake and Comparative Analysis

As the politicization of the pandemic grew, many researchers began examining how trust in science, exposure to and belief in conspiracy theories, and political ideology all combined in various forms to affect whether citizens planned to obtain a vaccination (Porteny et al., 2022). Many observed that the back-and-forth interactions from the Trump administration regarding the vaccine contributed to hesitation on the part of his Republican followers. Human clinical trials on vaccines began in March 2020 (Albrecht, 2022), and indeed, President Trump was quick to claim victory about this expedience (Romer & Jamieson, 2021). However, as delays occurred in receiving emergency approval and rolling out the vaccine, President Trump changed his stance and once again criticized the scientific community as being involved in a political conspiracy to slow down release to reduce his chance of a 2020 reelection (Romer & Jamieson, 2021).

Numerous studies examining vaccine uptake and intention highlight the connection between political ideology and vaccine receptivity and uptake. Indeed, studies consistently find that political conservatism (in the United States and other countries) reduces vaccine uptake (Albrecht, 2022). Specifically in the United States, researchers find that those who are Republicans, intend to vote for Donald Trump's re-election in 2020, or trust in the Whitehouse (which at the time reflected Donald Trump as president) consistently show a reduced intention for receiving a COVID-19 vaccine (Adhikari et al., 2022; Albrecht, 2022; Bolsen & Palm, 2022; Kreps & Kriner, 2021; Latkin et al., 2023; Lin et al., 2020; Porteny et al., 2022). Trying to disentangle the processes that underlie how political ideology shapes these intention behaviors is challenging, but most researchers suggest that political ideology serves as a lens to frame citizens understanding of trust (in science and government) and their perceived relationship between themselves and the state (Marien & Hooghe, 2011; St-Amant et al., 2021). To this burgeoning literature, I contend that like masks, vaccines also became a symbol representing a tripartite statement of one's willingness (or not) to trust in science, the media, and the government.

Given the abundance of data, I expect to find political party to be a significant predictor of intended vaccine uptake, with Republicans in the United States being less likely to report uptake intention and left-leaning parties in Finland being more likely to report uptake. I believe that political ideology became a forefront identity that shaped many citizens ideas about what the vaccines meant, not only as a preventative medicine to stop the spread of COVID-19, but as an important symbol that showed citizens willingness, or not, to partake in a measure that represented trust in science and the government. However, given our earlier findings that some collaborative dimensions remained significant predictors of compliance for mask wearing in November 2020, I also believe that some of them will show significance for intended vaccine uptake. While political leaders and media created a narrative that linked mask wearing and vaccine uptake as important symbols representing citizens' beliefs that those demands are scientifically fallible and governmentally intrusive on one side, or scientifically valid and governmentally legitimate on the other, the interactions between citizens and their governments that affect compliance run deep and are often about the perceived trust in those interactions (Levi & Stoker, 2000).

Thus, in an envisioned collaborative relationship between citizens and the state, citizens having access to information, understanding their role in combatting the pandemic, trusting fellow citizens to do their part, engaging in mutuality to do their own part for their communities and families, and acknowledging the challenges of compliance, can compel compliance to health-protective behaviors (Sedgwick et al., 2022). Despite revolving parties in power, the relationship between citizens and the state (particularly in Western Democratic nations) reflect belief in the fundamental institutions of a democracy (Inglehart, 1999). When citizens perceive these institutions as legitimate, they adopt the normative values of compliance with governmental requests because this is something they are expected to do (Dalton, 2004). To this point, when studying the outcomes of 33 nations in the European Values Survey, Marien and Hooghe (2011) find a robust significant negative relationship between political trust and legal permissiveness, indicating that as citizens report higher levels of political trust, they are

## 136  Donna Sedgwick

less likely to be permissive about citizens participating in illegal behaviors, such as cheating on taxes or claiming government benefits illegally.

Thus, as trust is an essential component of collaborative relationships (Sedgwick, 2017; Sedgwick et al., 2022; Thomson & Perry, 2006), when governments request that their citizens comply with mandates, citizens envision themselves, other citizens, and the government in a reciprocal relationship. When citizens acknowledge those collaborative dimensions, they take on those mandates as something they are expected to do and trust that other citizens are willing to do the same (Sedgwick et al., 2022). I argue that while political party may have become an important predictor for citizen's vaccine intention, those who still envision the citizen/state collaborative relationship, despite their political ideology, will be more likely to comply with vaccine receptivity. I turn now to a regression analysis of factors that affect vaccine intention for both US and Finnish residents in November 2020. In Table 8.3, I report the standardized betas and significance levels for panel samples of US and Finnish residents.

Table 8.3.   Factors That Affect Vaccine Intention, November 2020.

|  | The United States | Finland |
| --- | --- | --- |
| *Collaborative dimensions* | | |
| Understand role | 0.016 | 0.006 |
| Easily find information | 0.037 | –0.047 |
| COVID-19 guidelines easy to follow | 0.064 | 0.021 |
| Combat if everyone follows guidelines | 0.160** | –0.011 |
| Follow to protect myself/family | –0.170** | 0.085 |
| Follow to protect my community | 0.085 | 0.058 |
| Following guidelines are challenging | 0.016 | 0.079* |
| *Other factors* | | |
| Support political party in power | –0.087* | 0.120*** |
| Worry about COVID-19 | 0.159*** | 0.157*** |
| Social capital | 0.052 | 0.061 |
| Confidence in science | 0.119** | 0.179*** |
| *Controls* | | |
| Female | –0.150*** | –0.176*** |
| Age | 0.057 | 0.151*** |
| Married | –0.004 | –0.024 |
| College degree | 0.189*** | 0.046 |

$* p < 0.05; ** p < 0.01; *** p < 0.001.$

*Note*: All models are significant with RSQs ranging from 0.20 to 0.21.

Compliance with Protective Health Behaviors *137*

The findings from the regression analysis, see Table 8.3, reveal some expected and surprising results. Similar to earlier results, worry about COVID-19 remained a positive and strong predictor for vaccine intention. I also find that some controls were significant. For the United States, citizens with a college degree were more likely to report vaccine intention compared to those with less than a college degree. In Finland, older citizens intended to obtain a vaccination more than younger citizens. Perhaps surprising, but in line with other research on vaccine intention (see Lin et al., 2020), females in both the United States and Finland were less likely to report vaccine intention.

Some additional findings were also expected. As anticipated with the rise of significance of political party as a predictor for mask wearing, I also find it mattered for predicting vaccine intention for both US and Finnish citizens. Republicans in the United States were significantly less likely to report vaccine intention, whereas those Finnish residents who were members of left-leaning political parties were more likely to report vaccine intention. Also as expected, citizens in both countries that reported more confidence in science were more likely to plan on being vaccinated.

The collaborative dimension factors showed some similarities to the mask wearing analysis from November 2020 but also some surprising differences. For United States, citizens who call on all citizens to do their part to combat the pandemic were more likely to report vaccine intention. For Finnish residents, those citizens who reported that following the COVID-19 guidelines are challenging were also more likely to report vaccine intention. While this may seem counterintuitive, this finding is in line with Sedgwick et al. (2022), who argue that complying with challenging requests can indicate a commitment to the citizen/state relationship. Thus, at least one of the collaborative dimensions remains a positive predictor for both the United States and Finland.

However, a surprising finding is that US citizens who identified that they follow the guidelines to protect themselves and their families reported being *less likely* to obtain a vaccine. The mutuality dimension captures that people participate in collaborative relationships for their own benefits, but also for greater community benefits, and this self/family indicator highlights those personal benefits (Sedgwick et al., 2022). There are some possible explanations for this finding. First, it could be that those citizens who prioritize the benefits of compliance for themselves or their families were more influenced by concerns that were raised about the safety of the vaccine, primarily made popular by social media and conservative broadcast news. Additionally, agreeing to follow mandates to protect yourself or your family may highlight the tribalism aspects of the mutuality dimension by focusing on what is good for me and for my family. As nationalist leaders and conservative media exacerbated concerns about the safety of the vaccine, they were calling on their followers to not blindly partake in the vaccine but to protect their own tribe (Clark & Bain-Selbo, 2022). This finding highlights the delicate balance inherent in the mutuality aspect of collaboration; that is, when the parties involved in working toward a common goal begin to lose sight that "Us" contains not only immediate family and friends but also a greater community "Us," then outcomes similar to the Tragedy of the Commons may occur (Clark & Bain-Selbo, 2022).

## 138    *Donna Sedgwick*

However, the fact that those who believe that combatting the pandemic is possible if everyone follows the guidelines (for US residents) gives hope that there are still those, regardless of political ideology, who can still envision the social cohesion needed to come together for a collective good (Lofredo, 2020).

## Concluding Thoughts

The long-lasting effects of the pandemic are still revealing themselves across the globe. While many aspects of life have returned to normal, the findings from this study on the change in importance of political party and the diminishing (at least somewhat) of collaborative dimensions in predicting mask wearing and vaccine intention offer signs of mixed hope as citizens move forward and potentially face new and daunting challenges. On one hand, if the pandemic has taught us anything, political leaders who fuel polarization among their constituents result in negative outcomes for public health initiatives. Given the abundance of research on how political party mattered in determining whether someone followed the health-protective behaviors and intended to be vaccinated, our research findings are not surprising. As argued in this chapter, masks and vaccines became powerful symbols in a short amount of time that came to indicate to others whether they believed or questioned science, and if they agreed or not with health-protective behaviors in the name of public health. On the other hand, our findings from April 2020 show that political party *did not* matter for predicting mask wearing for either the United States or Finland. At that time, what mattered more was citizens being committed to their role in a citizen/state collaborative relationship to battle the pandemic together. Unfortunately, only seven months world leaders downplayed the importance of the larger "Us" and instead placed their attention on dividing interests. This finding suggests that political leaders and public health officials have a short amount of time to rally together and argue that indeed citizens are an "Us" when facing something as extreme as a pandemic if they wish to quell the spread of disease and move toward ending a pandemic.

## References

Adhikari, B., Cheah, P. Y., & von Seidlein, L. (2022). Trust is the common denominator for COVID-19 vaccine acceptance: A literature review. *Vaccine: 12*, 100213.

Albrecht, D. (2022). Vaccination, politics and COVID-19 impacts. *BMC Public Health, 22*(1), 1–12.

Alexander, M. (2012). *The new Jim crow* (Rev. ed.). The New Press.

Barry, C. L., Anderson, K. E., Han, H., Presskreischer, R., & McGinty, (2021). Change over time in public support for social distancing, mask wearing, and contact tracing to combat the COVID- 19 pandemic among US adults, April to November 2020. *American Journal of Public Health, 111*(5), 937–948.

Bernacer, J., García-Manglano, J., Camina, E., & Güell, F. (2021). Polarization of beliefs as a consequence of the COVID-19 pandemic: The case of Spain. *PloS One, 16*(7), e0254511.

Compliance with Protective Health Behaviors    139

Bierwiaczonek, K., Kunst, J. R., & Pich, O. (2020). Belief in COVID-19 conspiracy theories reduces social distancing over time. *Applied Psychology: Health and Well-Being*, *12*(4), 1270–1285.

Bish, A., & Michie, S. (2010). Demographic and attitudinal determinants of protective behaviours during a pandemic: A review. *British Journal of Health Psychology*, *15*(4), 797–824

Bolsen, T., & Palm, R. (2022). Politicization and COVID-19 vaccine resistance in the US. *Progress in Molecular Biology and Translational Science*, *188*(1), 81–100.

Blumer, H. (1969). *Symbolic interactionism: Perspective and method*. Prentice-Hall.

Braithwaite, J., & Makkai, T. (1994). Trust and compliance. *Policing and Society: An International Journal*, *4*(1), 1–12.

Brooks, J. T., & Butler, J. C. (2021). Effectiveness of mask wearing to control community spread of SARS-CoV-2. *Jama*, *325*(10), 998–999.

Burgess, A., & Horii, M. (2012). Risk, ritual and health responsibilisation: Japan's safety blanket of surgical face mask wearing. *Social Health Illness*, *34*(8), 1184–1198. https://doi.org/10.1111/j.1467-9566.2012.01466.x

Cava, M. A., Fay, K. E., Beanlands, H. J., McCay, E. A., & Wignall, R. (2005). Risk perception and compliance with quarantine during the SARS outbreak. *Journal of Nursing Scholarship*, *37*(4), 343–347.

Chuang, Y. C., Huang, Y. L., Tseng, K. C., Yen, C. H., & Yang, L. H. (2015). Social capital and health-protective behavior intentions in an influenza pandemic. *PloS One*, *10*(4), e0122970.

Clark, K. M., & Bain-Selbo, E. (2022). Tribalism and compassion in the age of a pandemic. *Soundings: An Interdisciplinary Journal*, *105*(2), 143–223.

Dada, S., Ashworth, H. C., Bewa, M. J., & Dhatt, R. (2021). Words matter: Political and gender analysis of speeches made by heads of government during the COVID-19 pandemic. *BMJ Global Health*, *6*(1), e003910.

Dalton, R. (2004). *Democratic challenges, democratic choices: The erosion of political support in advanced industrial democracies*. Oxford University Press.

Delen, D., Eryarsoy, E., & Davazdahemami, B. (2020). No place like home: Cross-national data analysis of the efficacy of social distancing during the COVID-19 pandemic. *JMIR Public Health and Surveillance*, *6*(2), e19862.

French, P. (2020, April 4). *In the 1918 flu pandemic, not wearing a mask was illegal in some parts of America. What changes?* CNN. https://www.cnn.com/2020/04/03/americas/flu-america-1918-masks-intl-hnk/index.html

Hao, F., Shao, W., & Huang, W. (2021). Understanding the influence of contextual factors and individual social capital on American public mask wearing in response to COVID-19. *Health & Place*, *68*, 102537

Hawdon, J. E. (2001). The role of presidential rhetoric in the creation of a moral panic: Reagan, Bush, and the war on drugs. *Deviant Behavior*, *22*(5), 419–445.

He, Z., & Chen, Z. (2021). The social group distinction of nationalists and globalists amid COVID-19 pandemic. *Fudan Journal of the Humanities and Social Sciences*, *14*(1), 67–85.

Im, T., Cho, W., Porumbescu, G., & Park, J. (2014). Internet, trust in government, and citizen compliance. *Journal of Public Administration Research and Theory*, *24*(3), 741–763.

Inglehart, R. (1999). Postmodernization erodes respect for authority, but increases support for democracy. In P. Norris (Ed.), *Critical citizens: Global support for democratic government* (pp. 236–256). Oxford University Press.

Jacobs, P., & Ohinmaa, A. P. (2020). The enforcement of statewide mask wearing mandates to prevent COVID-19 in the US: an overview. *F1000Research*, *9*, 1–11.

Kang, K. E., Vedlitz, A., Goldsmith, C. L., & Seavey, I. (2023). Optimism and pessimism toward science: A new way to look at the public's evaluations of science and

## 140 Donna Sedgwick

technology discoveries and recommendations. *Politics and the Life Sciences*, *42*(2), 234–253.

Koivula, A., Räsänen, P., Marttila, E., Sedgwick, D., & Hawdon, J. (2023). COVID-19 compliance and media consumption: A longitudinal study of Finland and the US during the first year of COVID-19. *Journal of Broadcasting & Electronic Media*, *67*(4), 530–552.

Koljonen, J., & Palonen, E. (2021). Performing COVID-19 control in Finland: Interpretative topic modelling and discourse theoretical reading of the government communication and hashtag landscape. *Frontiers in Political Science*, *3*, 689614.

Koskan, A. M., Teeter, B. S., Daniel, C. L., LoCoco, I. E., Jensen, U. T., & Ayers, S. L. (2023). US adults' reasons for changing their degree of willingness to vaccinate against COVID-19. *Journal of Public Health*, *32*(3), 355–367.

Kreps, S. E., & Kriner, D. L. (2021). Factors influencing Covid-19 vaccine acceptance across subgroups in the United States: Evidence from a conjoint experiment. *Vaccine*, *39*(24), 3250–3258.

Latkin, C., Dayton, L., Miller, J., Eschliman, E., Yang, J., Jamison, A., & Kong, X. (2023). Trusted information sources in the early months of the COVID-19 pandemic predict vaccination uptake over one year later. *Vaccine*, *41*(2), 573–580.

Levi, M., & Stoker, L. (2000). Political trust and trustworthiness. *Annual Review of Political Science*, *3*(1), 475–507.

Lin, C., Tu, P., & Beitsch, L. M. (2020). Confidence and receptivity for COVID-19 vaccines: A rapid systematic review. *Vaccines*, *9*(1), 16.

Lindholm, J., Carlsson, T., Albrecht, F., & Hermansson, H. (2023). Communicating Covid-19 on social media: Analysing the use of Twitter and Instagram by Nordic health authorities and prime ministers. In B. Johansson, Ø. Ihlen, J. Lindholm, & M. Blach-Ørsten (Eds.), *Communicating a pandemic: Crisis management and Covid-19 in the Nordic countries* (pp. 149–172). University of Gothenburg. https://doi.org/10.48335/9789188855688-7

Lofredo, M. P. (2020). Social cohesion, trust, and government action against pandemics. *Eubios Journal of Asian and International Bioethics*, *30*(4), 182–189.

Lupton, D., Southerton, C., Clark, M., & Watson, A. (2021). *The face mask in COVID times: A sociomaterial analysis*. De Gruyter.

Marien, S., & Hooghe, M. (2011). Does political trust matter? An empirical investigation into the relation between political trust and support for law compliance. *European Journal of Political Research*, *50*(2), 267–291.

Mead, G. H. (1934). *Mind, self, & society*. University of Chicago Press.

Morrison, C. (2020, June 3). *Stay at home orders give way to curfews*. Washington Examiner. https://www.washingtonexaminer.com/news/2611809/stay-at-home-orders-give-way-to-curfews/

Nocera, J., & McLean, B. (2023). *The big fail: What the pandemic revealed about who America protects and who it leaves behind*. Penguin.

Pearce, K. (2020, March 13). What is social distancing and how can it slow the spread of Covid-19? *Hub. Johns Hopkins University*. https://hub.jhu.edu/2020/03/13/what-is-social-distancing/

Porteny, T., Corlin, L., Allen, J. D., Monahan, K., Acevedo, A., Stopka, T. J., Levine, P., & Ladin, K. (2022). Associations among political voting preference, high-risk health status, and preventative behaviors for COVID-19. *BMC Public Health*, *22*(1), 1–9.

Prati, G., Pietrantoni, L., & Zani, B. (2011). Compliance with recommendations for pandemic influenza H1N1 2009: The role of trust and personal beliefs. *Health Education Research*, *26*(5), 761–769.

Quinn, S. C., Kumar, S., Freimuth, V. S., Kidwell, K., & Musa, D. (2009). Public willingness to take a vaccine or drug under emergency use authorization during the 2009 H1N1 pandemic. *Biosecurity and Bioterrorism: Biodefense Strategy, Practice, and Science,* 7(3), 275–290.

Ren, J., & Feagin, J. (2021). Face mask symbolism in anti-Asian hate crimes. *Ethnic and Racial Studies, 44*(5), 746–758.

Richards, I. (2022). Neoliberalism, COVID-19 and conspiracy: pandemic management strategies and the far-right social turn. *Justice, Power and Resistance, 5*(1–2), 109–126.

Romer, D., & Jamieson, K. H. (2021). Conspiratorial thinking, selective exposure to conservative media, and response to COVID-19 in the US. *Social Science & Medicine, 291*, 114480.

Rubin, G. J., Amlôt, R., Page, L., & Wessely, S. (2009). Public perceptions, anxiety, and behaviour change in relation to the swine flu outbreak: cross sectional telephone survey. *BMJ, 339*, 1–8.

Sedgwick, D. (2017). Building collaboration: Examining the relationship between collaborative processes and activities. *Journal of Public Administration Research and Theory, 27*(2), 236–252.

Sedgwick, D., Hawdon, J., Räsänen, P., & Koivula, A. (2022). The role of collaboration in complying with COVID-19 health protective behaviors: A cross-national study. *Administration & Society, 54*(1), 29–56.

St-Amant, O., Parada, H., & Wilson-Mitchell, K. (2021). The COVID-19 mask: Toward an understanding of social meanings and responses. *Advances in Nursing Science, 45*(2), 100–113.

Tang, C., & Wong, C. (2003). An outbreak of severe acute respiratory syndrome: Predictors of health behaviors and effect of community prevention measures in Hong Kong, China. *American Journal of Public Health, 93*(11), 1887–1188.

Thomson, A. M., & Perry, J. L. (2006). Collaboration processes: Inside the black box. *Public Administration Review, 66*, 20–32.

Travaglino, G. A., & Moon, C. (2021). Compliance and self-reporting during the COVID-19 pandemic: A cross-cultural study of trust and self-conscious emotions in the United States, Italy, and South Korea. *Frontiers in Psychology, 12*, 565845.

Van Rooij, B., de Bruijn, A. L., Reinders Folmer, C., Kooistra, E. B., Kuiper, M. E., Brownlee, M., Olthuis, E., & Fine, A. (2020). *Compliance with COVID-19 mitigation measures in the United States* [Research paper 2020-21]. Amsterdam Law School.

Vos, J. (2021). *The psychology of COVID-19: building resilience for future pandemics* (1st ed.). SAGE.

Vosoughi, S., Roy, D., & Aral, S. (2018). The spread of true and false news online. *American Association for the Advancement of Science, 359*(6380), 1146–1151.

# Chapter 9

# The Pandemic's Effects in Finland and the United States: The Long-term Consequences of Early Perceptions and Behaviors

*James Hawdon and Donna Sedgwick*

*Virginia Tech, USA*

### Abstract

This chapter weaves the finding from the previous chapters together to explain how perceptions of and responses to a pandemic are not static but change over the course of the pandemic and in between the governance and social welfare structures of the nations they affect. We consider the cross-national differences in outcomes and relate these to a variety of strategies used to curb the pandemic's spread. We then conduct a series of analyses that examine our underlying arguments using data collected in November 2023, approximately 6 months after the pandemic was declared to be over. We find that compliance with health-protective recommendations is correlated with positive health outcomes. Specifically, we investigate how compliance correlates with the number of times an individual became ill with COVID-19. We then use variables discussed throughout the book to investigate how these factors correlate with complying with protective health measures, including being vaccinated and wearing face coverings during the pandemic. We find that collaborative factors are good predictors of compliance with health-protective recommendations. We then investigate how factors such as planned behavioral changes to mitigate the pandemic's effect, attitudes toward government spending, media consumption, political party, and exposure to hate materials relate to the compliance factors. Ultimately, we demonstrate how the behavior of elites and the perceptions

---

Perceptions of a Pandemic: A Cross-Continental Comparison of Citizen Perceptions, Attitudes, and Behaviors During COVID-19, 143–168
Copyright © 2025 by James Hawdon and Donna Sedgwick
Published under exclusive licence by Emerald Publishing Limited
doi:10.1108/978-1-83608-624-620241009

## 144  *James Hawdon and Donna Sedgwick*

and attitudes of citizens during the initial stages of the pandemic shaped the pandemic's long-term consequences. The chapter concludes by summarizing the findings from the previous chapters to set the stage for the concluding chapter.

*Keywords*: Confidence in institutions; collaborative relationships; compliance with health mandates; COVID-19-related illness; COVID-19 and well-being

# Introduction

Estimating the total cost of the COVID-19 pandemic is nearly impossible. As of March 2024, it is estimated that people contracted over 700 million cases of the virus and over 7 million people (almost 2 million more than the population of Finland and about twice the population of Oklahoma) died from it (Worldometer, 2024, March 26). In addition to the horrendous loss of human life, it is estimated that over 65 million people continue to struggle with the debilitating post-infection effects of "long COVID" (Lancet, 2023). While the loss of life and additional health complications associated with the virus are the most significant consequences of the pandemic, it also wreaked havoc on the world's economy. The costs associated with workplace absences, loss of retail in traditional stores, decreased travel, closing of public spaces, increased healthcare costs, mandated and voluntary lockdowns, and disruptions to the global supply chain are staggering. By mid-2023, the pandemic's cost to the US economy alone was over $14 trillion (Halávka & Rose, 2023). The loss to the nation's gross domestic product was twice that experienced during the Great Recession of 2007–2009 and 20 times greater than the economic costs associated with the 9/11 terrorist attacks (Halávka & Rose, 2023). Of course, these estimates are multiplied many times over when applied at the global level. Moreover, these estimates do not consider the emotional toll, the loss of educational opportunities, the global increase in inequality, or the heightened political polarization related to the COVID-19 pandemic. Although scholars may quibble over how to accurately measure cases, deaths, and costs of the pandemic, it was unquestionably devastating to many. In fact, it was undoubtedly the most devastating and tragic event humanity has collectively faced since World War II.

Taking a narrower view of the costs of COVID-19 by considering the two nations focused on throughout this book, a pattern emerges. The United States accounted for the most COVID-19 cases worldwide, with over 111 million reported cases. The United States also had the highest number of deaths with over 1.2 million Americans dying from the virus. By comparison, Finland reported 1.5 million cases and slightly less than 12,000 deaths. Given the nations' difference in population, these numbers are unsurprising. However, comparing the two nations more directly, the United States reported 333,719 cases per million population while Finland reported 272,900 cases per million population. The United States also had a higher death rate from the virus. The United States had the

Pandemic's Effects in Finland and the United States **145**

14th highest death rate at 3,639 deaths per million population while Finland ranked 52nd with a rate of 2,153 deaths per million population (Worldometer, 2024, March 26). Regardless of the controversy over how to count COVID-19-related deaths, the United States fared poorly despite its relative wealth and advanced medical system. This relative toll suffered by the citizens of the United States is true not only in comparison to Finland, but in comparison to most nations. Comparatively, Finland fared better than the United States, and it also fared better than many of its European neighbors. The purpose of this chapter is to ask the question "why." What can we learn from our data to help make sense of the virus's relatively high toll in the United States? How did the American and Finnish responses to the onset of the virus contribute to the different outcomes these nations experienced? And, most importantly, how do these insights help us better prepare for the next pandemic or similar crisis?

## Early Perceptions and Long-term Consequences

As the previous chapters argued, the perceptions and behaviors we had and performed at the beginning of the pandemic had long-term consequences. Some of those ideas and behaviors turned out to be unnecessary but harmless. Remember carefully bringing in the mail and leaving it unopened for several days? Remember wearing gloves while filling up the gas tank? Remember cleaning and disinfecting frequently handled objects? With hindsight, we can say these behaviors did not prevent one from getting COVID-19, but they certainly did not harm anyone.

Other behaviors some people engaged in were unnecessary and harmful. Remember when former President Trump suggested the White House Coronavirus Task Force investigate injecting disinfectant at the site of the infection? This suggestion turned out to be dangerous advice as accidental poisonings increased after the president's comments (Kluger, 2020; also see Rivera et al., 2020). Remember when some advocated developing "herd immunity" instead of social distancing? While it is debated, it appears that strategy was costly in terms of lives. For example, Sweden, the nation that pursued the strategy most openly, had far higher COVID-19-related death rates than did the other Scandinavian nations. Sweden's rate was 2,680 per million population while Finland's (2,153), Denmark's (1,511), Norway's (1,204), and Iceland's (663) were considerably lower (see Worldometer, 2024, March 26).

Other actions had very mixed effects. Remember the anti-parasite medicine Ivermectin? This medicine turned out to help some, but also was dangerous for others. Research demonstrated that Ivermectin was ineffective at preventing COVID-19, hospitalization from the virus, or mortality, although it may have reduced the need for mechanical ventilation and other adverse events (see Abd-Elsalam et al., 2021; Popp et al., 2021; Reis et al., 2022; Song et al., 2024). While Ivermectin may have had some benefits, it also became the focus of the anti-vaccine movement (Huang, 2021), which implicates it in numerous unnecessary deaths. Other earlier perceptions, behaviors, and recommendations were similarly confusing and potentially harmful. Remember being told not to wear face coverings so they could be saved for doctors and nurses, but then strongly encouraged to wear them? Remember being told it was relatively safe to gather

## 146    James Hawdon and Donna Sedgwick

in small groups? Some said fewer than 50 while others said no more than 10. Not only was the contradictory advice about the size of the group confusing, but it also turns out that it only takes one infected person to pass on the SARS-CoV-2 virus. Thus, gathering with others, regardless of the size of the group, was potentially dangerous if the group included an infected person.

Other early perceptions – such as the deadly seriousness of the disease – helped convince people to take necessary precautions. Similarly, other behaviors that some of us adopted in the initial stages of the pandemic – such as social distancing and mask wearing – turned out to be both necessary and lifesaving (see, e.g., Ford et al., 2021; Hansen & Mano, 2023; Lyu & Wehby, 2020). Other attitudes – such as supporting the $18 billion investment in developing vaccines – turned out to be vitally important in saving lives and ending the pandemic.

Thus, our early perceptions and behaviors were varied, and some had dramatic consequences while others did not. But can variations in the perceptions and behaviors between Americans and Finns that are captured in our data help explain the differential effects of the virus in the two nations? We believe they can. Ultimately, the critical question is if the differences in early perceptions and behaviors mattered in terms of well-being, sickness, and lost lives. Let us begin answering that question by considering national-level data then turning to our data that consider the relationship between complying with health-protective behaviors as recommended by the governments and leading health organizations of the two nations. We will then work backwards to investigate what likely led to complying with those recommendations and considering how these factors varied in the two nations.

## Health Recommendations and Health Outcomes

As noted above, COVID-19 outcomes were worse in the United States than they were in Finland. This is true in terms of both rates of illness and rates of death. In terms of available secondary data, these differing outcomes can be attributed to differing rates of compliance with several health mandates.

### Vaccines

Of course, the primary factor that saved lives was the development of effective, life-saving vaccines. For example, at a local level, research suggests that the vaccines saved over 48,000 hospitalizations and 8,000 deaths in New York City just by helping reduce the spread of the Alpha and Delta variants in the spring of 2021 (Shoukat et al., 2022). At a broader scale, it is estimated that between 140,000 and 232,000 lives were saved in the United States by early spring 2021 (see Gupta et al., 2021; Jia et al., 2023), and nearly 750,000 lives were saved through June 2023 (Atkeson, 2023). Comparable results were found in Europe, where it is estimated that vaccinations reduced deaths in Europe by 57% and saved at least 1.4 million lives (Mesle et al., 2024). Worldwide, it is estimated that the staggered rollout of vaccines across 141 countries prevented over 2.4 million excess deaths (Agrawal et al., 2023). In short, the vaccines saved lives and were instrumental in ending the pandemic, and Finns were more likely to be vaccinated than

*Pandemic's Effects in Finland and the United States* **147**

were Americans. For example, based on data from *Our World in Data*, by November 2022, 81.6% of Finns and 80.2% of Americans were partially vaccinated. While these differences are not striking, the national differences become greater when we consider the number of people partially vaccinated and boosted. While 78.4% of Finns were fully vaccinated and 72.9% had received at least one booster shot, only 68.5% of Americans were fully vaccinated and only 42.6% had been boosted. In total, as of mid-2023, Finland administered 238.5 doses of the vaccine per 100 people compared to the United States' 203.8 doses per 100 people (Our World in Data, 2024a).

Our third wave of data, collected after the pandemic was declared over in November 2023, reflects similar differences in vaccinations between the two nations. First, respondents were asked if they had received a COVID-19 vaccination. Over 86% of Finnish respondents (1,380 of 1,599 respondents) answered the question affirmatively, while only 72.4% (1,142) of the 1,578 American respondents did so. We also asked if they had received a COVID-19 booster. The overwhelming majority of Finnish respondents had been boosted, with 30.2% receiving one and 51.0% receiving two or more boosters. Only 81 of 1,380 (5.9%) Finnish respondents who had been vaccinated at all did not get boosted. The US respondents provide a stark contrast. Among American respondents who were vaccinated, a full 261 (or 22.9%) had not been boosted at all. Only 32.0% were boosted once, and an additional 46.2% had been boosted two or more times. Thus, similar to the available secondary data, our data show that not only were Finns more likely to protect themselves with one vaccination, but they were also far more likely to be boosted. Based on these data alone and the evidence regarding the importance of the vaccine in saving lives, it is understandable why the COVID-19-related death rate was higher in the United States than it was in Finland.

Our data also indicate that vaccines helped not only save lives, but they also reduced the likelihood of becoming ill. We asked respondents, "How many times, if any, have you had COVID?" Responses to this item were "none," "once," "twice," three times," "four or more times," "I have had it, but I am unsure how many times," and "I am unsure if I ever had COVID." Recoding those who said they had it but were unsure of how many times they had it as having it "twice" and those who were unsure if they ever had COVID-19 as missing, we then correlate this variable with if they had been vaccinated. We find that the correlation was inverse and significant in both countries. In the United States, being vaccinated at all was inversely related with the number of times one became ill ($r = -0.054$; $p = 0.037$), as was being boosted ($r = -0.073$; $p = 0.005$). In Finland, being vaccinated was inversely related to number of times one was ill ($r = -0.015$), but this was not statistically significant ($p = 0.567$). However, being boosted was significantly related to the number of times one became ill ($r = -0.119$; $p < 0.01$).[1]

---

[1]We also analyzed the relationship using different coding schemes for those who did not know the number of times they had COVID-19 or if they ever had COVID-19. While the strength of the correlations changed, all coding schemes produced similar substantive results. In short, getting vaccinated reduced the likelihood of becoming ill.

## 148  *James Hawdon and Donna Sedgwick*

The lack of significance for solely being vaccinated is likely due to the lack of variation in vaccination status among Finnish respondents as 86% of them were vaccinated. Similarly, recoding the variable as a dichotomous variable that compared those who had COVID-19 with those who never had it produced similar results: those who were boosted were less likely to have ever been sick with COVID-19 ($r = -0.050$; $p = 0.049$ and $r = -0.093$; $p < 0.001$ in the United States and Finland, respectively). While these correlations are modest, we need to remember that those who were not vaccinated, contracted COVID-19, and subsequently passed away because of the disease were not included in this sample. Including those individuals would have undoubtedly strengthened the correlation. Consequently, the vaccines mattered both in terms of saving lives and in terms of reducing the chances of becoming ill. This is another piece of evidence that supports the efficacy of the various COVID-19 vaccinations.

### Other Mitigation Efforts

While differences in the vaccination rates between the two nations likely account for the majority of the differential health outcomes, we are interested in the early health-protective behaviors adopted in the two nations and if these can help explain the variation in outcomes. Evidence suggests that actions to mitigate the effects of the pandemic early helped save lives by slowing its spread. Lockdowns, while far more costly than the vaccines and not without their own problems, also saved lives (see Arbel & Pliskin, 2022; Cerqueti et al., 2022; Miles et al., 2021; Yakusheva et al., 2022). Similarly, wearing masks, especially high-quality masks, also likely reduced the loss of life (see Andrejko, 2022; Chu et al., 2020; Enright et al., 2024; Hansen & Mano, 2023; Howard et al., 2021; Lyu & Wehby, 2020; contrast Spira, 2022). Other mitigation efforts, such as social distancing, also helped save lives (Chu et al., 2020). These mitigation efforts significantly contributed to slowing the spread of the virus. In fact, it is likely that the vaccines, as important as they were, would have come along too late to save significant numbers of lives had these early mitigation efforts been completely relaxed (see Atkeson, 2023). So, what does the evidence say about how Americans and Finns did adopting these early strategies?

### Contact Tracing and Testing

There is some secondary evidence that suggests that Finland engaged in some early behaviors that mattered. For example, Finland implemented full "comprehensive contact tracing" while the United States only did "limited contact tracing" (Our World in Data, 2024b). Finland also made testing more widely available than did the United States. Contact tracing combined with effective testing was found to reduce the spread of COVID-19. For example, in a systematic review of 14 observational and modeling studies, all showed consistent evidence, albeit with low certainty, that contact tracing was associated with better COVID-19 control (Juneau et al., 2023).

*Pandemic's Effects in Finland and the United States* **149**

This could explain the different infection rates in the two nations in the initial stages of the pandemic. Likely due to the widespread availability of testing, Finland experienced an initial spike of almost 30% of the population testing positive in March, after which the daily positive COVID-19 tests dropped to below 10% of the population by the end of March. This relatively low rate was likely due to the comprehensive contact tracing. In the United States, the daily rate of positive tests began around 10% and spiked at about 20% in April. Unlike Finland, the rates of new positive tests in the United States continued to maintain about 5–15% throughout the remainder of 2020. Although these spikes probably represent an influx of testing rather than infection itself, it appears Finland was able to control rates of positive tests in 2020 better than the United States, which maintained a consistent rate of infection throughout that first year. Unfortunately, we do not have items in our data that can speak to these mitigation strategies, but it is likely that these measures helped slow the pandemic more effectively in Finland than in the United States.

## Face Coverings

Although Finland did better at contact tracing, the United States moved more quickly to require face coverings than did Finland, and Americans were required to wear face coverings longer than were Finns. While the United States recommended the use of face coverings as early as mid-March 2020 and moved to requiring face coverings outside the home by April 2020, Finland did not recommend using masks until August 2020. In March 2021, Finland moved to requiring face coverings in some public places, but this requirement only lasted until August 2021. Conversely, the United States maintained the requirement for wearing face coverings until May of that year when the requirement was relaxed to apply only to public places, and it was not until July 2021 that the United States moved to requiring masks only in some public places (Our World in Data, 2024c). Despite the United States requiring face coverings for much of the pandemic while Finland only recommended them for most of the pandemic, our data reveal little difference in overall wearing of masks. We asked our respondents in November 2023, "Thinking back to the pandemic, how likely were you to wear a mask when in public." As can be seen in Fig. 9.1, there is virtually no difference between the two nations in terms of the percentages that never wore a mask, rarely wore a mask, or only wore a mask sometimes. Finns were more likely than Americans to report wearing a mask "most of the times," while Americans reported wearing a mask "always or almost always" more than Finns did. However, when you combine these responses, 76.7% of Americans and 74.2% of Finns reported at least wearing a mask "most of the times."[2]

---

[2]The difference in mask wearing is not statistically significant when the variable is collapsed in this manner ($\chi^2 = 2.70$; $p = 0.100$).

150  James Hawdon and Donna Sedgwick

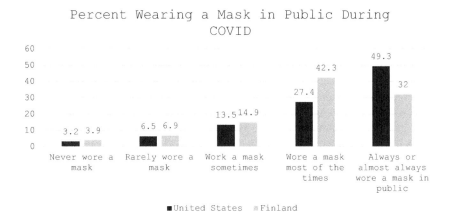

Fig. 9.1. Percent of Respondents Who Wore a Mask in Public During COVID-19.

Interestingly, while there is convincing evidence that masked helped curb the spread of COVID-19, eased the burden on hospitals, and ultimately saved lives (see Andrejko, 2022; Chu et al., 2020; Enright et al., 2024; Hansen & Mano, 2023; Howard et al., 2021; Lyu & Wehby, 2020), our data do not reflect this, at least in terms of becoming ill. The correlation between how often respondents wore a mask and the number of times they became ill with COVID-19 failed to approach statistical significance in either country. Of course, we need to remember that these correlations may be weaker than what would have been the case due to not including respondents who contracted COVID-19 and died from the disease. We also need to remember that the item we used asked people to recall their behaviors, and there are always problems with recalling behaviors accurately. This recall bias lowers the reliability of the question, which can only lower its predictive power. Nevertheless, our data do not suggest that requiring masks or wearing them reduced the number of times our respondents became ill with COVID-19.

*Restrictions and Shutdowns*

Next, the United States engaged in more restrictive actions when it came to shutdowns and restrictions. While both nations restricted internal movement for some, the United States required mandatory shutdowns for everyone except essential workers while Finland only recommended shutdowns. If we compare the "Government Stringency Index,"[3] which is a composite measure of how strict

---

[3]The stringency index is calculated based on the following nine policy metrics: school closures; workplace closures; cancelation of public events; restrictions on public gatherings; closures of public transport; stay-at-home requirements; public information campaigns; restrictions on internal movements; international travel controls (Our World in Data, 2024b).

*Pandemic's Effects in Finland and the United States* **151**

a policy response of a government is across nine policy measures (see Our World in Data, 2024d), the initial response by the Finnish government was relatively strict, reaching 71.3 out of 100 at the beginning of the pandemic in early April 2020. These restrictions were then relaxed relatively quickly, dropping to 32.3 by fall 2020. They were then toughened to 52.31 during the Delta wave of late fall 2020/winter 2021 before being relaxed again in the spring of 2021, with only a modest strengthening during the Omicron wave. By comparison, the stringency index reached a similar level in the United States at the initial stages of the pandemic at a slightly higher 72.69; however, it remained near 70 for the remainder of 2020 and through spring 2021. The index then remained consistently high in a relative sense, not reaching a low like Finland's 32.3 until August 2022 when it was 34.26 (Our World in Data, 2024d). Thus, based on these data, the United States implemented stricter governmental policies than did Finland. It should be noted that the strictness of these policies may have or may not have influenced transmission rates as their efficacy is debatable. In addition, as discussed throughout the text, the pandemic appears to have been more widespread in the United States than in Finland. If this is indeed true, the relative strictness of the governmental responses may have been appropriate to the level of risk that the pandemic posed to the community. Keeping these caveats in mind, these secondary data do not offer much help in terms of explaining the national differences in the health and well-being of the citizenry as these relate to the pandemic.

What these restrictions were meant to do was to limit citizens from interacting with people outside their family or network of close friends – what people began to referring to as "their pod." Our data provide evidence that most people did practice some forms of social distancing during the pandemic. For example, recalling the discussion in Chapter 2, Finnish respondents planned to alter their interactions with friends and families more so than Americans did, while Americans planned to change their consuming behaviors more so than Finns did. As it turned out, most people enacted their plans, but perhaps not as much as they had hoped. Using our 2023 data, close to 70% of Americans and 62% of Finns reported canceling plans to meet friends or family members because of COVID-19, which is reversed from our earlier findings. However, Americans did alter their consuming behaviors more so than did Finns. While 77% of Americans avoided busy public places during the pandemic, only 68% of Finns did so. Similarly, just under 70% of Americans stocked up on food and other necessities, but only 38% of Finnish respondents did so. Despite these national differences, however, there is evidence that early ideas about how to mitigate the virus's effect influenced the behaviors people chose to follow, just as the Theory of Planned Behavior would predict. Unfortunately, these practices did not appear to decrease the likelihood of the respondents becoming ill. In fact, the correlation between canceling plans with family or friends is positive and significant in both nations ($r = 0.149$; $p < 0.001$ and $r = 0.165$; $p < 0.001$ in the United States and Finland, respectively). These positive correlations undoubtedly indicate that those who got sick canceled plans rather than canceling plans led one to become ill, but the fact remains that our data do not indicate that – at least among our respondents – social distancing kept one from becoming ill with

## 152    James Hawdon and Donna Sedgwick

the virus (also see Nocera & McLean (2023) for a discussion of how lockdowns failed to prevent illness and deaths).

Consequently, reviewing the secondary data and the data we collected after the pandemic was over in November 2023 reveal that the vaccines helped reduce the odds of becoming ill. Other strategies, such as contact tracing, mask wearing, shutdowns, and social distancing, likely helped slow the spread of the disease, but these may not have prevented people from contracting the virus, at least among those who responded to our survey. As noted, the correlations we see in our data very well may be lower than what would have been observed if we were able to collect data on those who died from the virus, but among our respondents, only the vaccine and being boosted mattered.

## What Predicts Being Vaccinated?

Given the importance of the vaccines for preventing serious illness and death, it is important to discern what patterned who got a vaccine and who got a vaccine booster. To ascertain this information, we conducted logistic regression analyses predicting vaccinations and then if they were boosted. Relying primarily on collaboration theory as discussed in the last chapter and elsewhere (Sedgwick et al., 2022), we use a measure of collaboration and other factors to predict if the respondent was vaccinated and boosted. According to collaboration theory, the relationship between the state and its citizens can be understood as a collaborative partnership for the purpose of co-producing governance (Kathi & Cooper, 2005; Sedgwick, 2017; Thomson & Perry, 2006; Vigoda, 2002). That is, a partnership is formed where both governments and their citizenry have responsibilities to each other. In general, research suggests that those citizens who view the state as being a collaborative partner are more likely to comply with state mandates, including recommendations about health-protective behaviors (Aschhoff & Vogel, 2019; Sedgwick et al., 2022).

While our earlier surveys included several variables that tapped the various dimensions of collaboration theory (e.g., governance, administration, norms of trust, mutuality, and autonomy; see Sedgwick et al., 2022), our third wave of data included only single items that tapped each of these various dimensions. We had to revise the items to adjust for the fact that the pandemic had ended by the time the data were collected. Respondents were asked the extent to which they agreed with the following five-point Likert questions:

- I understand my roles and responsibilities as a citizen of Finland/United States.
- I can find information easily about government laws, agencies, or programs.
- The COVID-19 health (prevention) guidelines were clear for me to follow.
- We will be able to combat a national emergency or crisis if everyone follows government-issued guidelines and regulations.
- During a national crisis, I would follow government-issued guidelines to protect myself or family.
- During a national crisis, I would follow government-issued guidelines to protect my community.

Pandemic's Effects in Finland and the United States  **153**

These items were factor analyzed and were found to load on one dimension in both nations. Since the factor loading scores were similar across nations, we constructed the variable on the entire sample of both nations.[4] We also include a measure of social capital, but this variable was measured using the same items that were used in the earlier analyses (see the Appendix for items and operationalization of the concept of social capital).

In addition to forming a collaborative relationship with the state, the confidence citizens have in various institutions can influence if they comply with governmental recommendations and mandates (e.g., Badman et al., 2022; Bornstein & Tomkins, 2015; Shanka & Menebo, 2022). Similarly, in our data collected in 2020, respondents were asked if they would say they had a great deal of confidence, only some confidence, or hardly any confidence at all in the people who were running various institutions. For this analysis, we include the variables (1) confidence in the scientific community, (2) confidence in the federal government, (3) confidence in medicine or health care, and (4) confidence in the media.

Since people are more likely to comply with governmental requests if they are coming from the party or coalition they favor, we also include a measure of political party in the analyses. As in the earlier data, we code this as "the party in power" at the time of the pandemic. In the United States, the variable was coded as Republican versus Democrats, Independents, and others. This reflects that Donald Trump was president when the pandemic began and for the first year of pandemic. Although the Democratic Biden administration assumed power in January 2021 and held it throughout the remainder of the pandemic and while we collected the third wave of data, we retain the same coding as in earlier chapters for this analysis. We do the same for Finland, defining the ruling coalition as consisting of the Social Democratic Party, the Centre Party, the Green League, the Left Alliance, and the "Swedish People's Party." All other parties were coded as being in the opposition party.

As discussed in earlier chapters, media consumption and exposure to online hate can also influence how one views the government and therefore compliance. We construct a measure of omnivorous media consumption – those who consumed several different forms of media – by combining if the respondent watched television, read print media, or read online news or periodicals. The composite measure ranged from 0 (did not use any of these media) to 3 (used all of these media). We also include our measure of exposure to online hate that asked respondents "during the past 3 months, have you seen hateful or degrading writing or speech online inappropriately attacking individuals or groups." We also control for sex, age, and how worried they are about COVID-19.

---

[4]The one-factor solution produced an eigen-value of 3.14 and accounted for 52.9% of the variance in the six items. The factor loadings were roles and responsibilities (0.576), find information easily (0.549), guidelines were clear to follow (0.681), can combat national emergency if everyone follows governmental guidelines (0.789), I would follow guidelines to protect myself and my family (0.841), and during a crisis I would follow governmental guidelines (0.846).

## 154 James Hawdon and Donna Sedgwick

## Results

The first notable result is the within-nation consistency between the models predicting if the respondent was vaccinated and if the respondent received at least one booster. This is unsurprising in Finland since virtually everyone who received a vaccine also received a booster, but there were a considerable number of Americans who received only one vaccine. Still, the only differences between the vaccination and boosted model in Finland is that confidence in the media was a significant predictor of being boosted but not of getting a vaccine. The only differences between these models in the United States is that being worried about the pandemic significantly predicted being boosted but not receiving the initial vaccine, and males were more likely than females to be vaccinated initially, but there was no difference between males and females in terms of being boosted.

A second notable result is that the measure of viewing the citizen–state relationship as collaborative significantly predicted both being vaccinated and being boosted in both Finland and the United States. Confidence in the medical institution also was a significant predictor of both vaccination status and being boosted in both nations. Political party was also a significant predictor of being vaccinated and boosted in the United States, and it was a significant predictor of vaccination status and approached significance for being boosted in ($p = 0.059$) in Finland. The direction of this relationship was different when comparing the two nations. In Finland, being part of the left-leaning ruling coalition increased the odds of complying with the governmental recommendation to be vaccinated but being in the right-leaning ruling party in the United States (i.e., Republican) was inversely related to compliance. Of course, what this means is that across both nations, the more liberal one's political leaning, the greater the probability they complied with the recommendations to be vaccinated and boosted.

Therefore, several factors were consistent across models and between nations; however, there were some notable differences between the two nations. Given the similarities between the models, we will focus on the models predicting initial vaccination. Results for both nations are reported in Table 9.1.

In the United States, the model performed relatively well (–2 log likelihood = 1560.96, Naglkerke $R^2 = 0.250$).[5] As mentioned above, believing the relationship between the citizen and the state should be a collaborative partnership increased the odds of being vaccinated by 38%. Social solidarity, confidence in the medical institution, and confidence in the scientific community also increased the chances

---

[5]Collaborative dimensions (OR = 1.38; $p < 0.001$; CI 1.197–1.588); social solidarity (OR = 1.04; $p = 0.047$; CI 1.000–1.082); confidence in the medical institution (OR = 1.66; $p < 0.001$; CI 1.197–1.588); confidence in the scientific community (OR = 1.50; $p < 0.001$; CI 1.199–1.865); age (OR = 1.027; $p < 0.001$; CI 1.019–1.036); male (OR = 1.31; $p = 0.036$; CI 1.018–1.686); online hate exposure (OR = 1.48; $p = 0.004$; CI 1.134–1.897); Republican (OR = 0.54; $p < 0.001$; CI 0.406–0.709).

Pandemic's Effects in Finland and the United States    155

Table 9.1.    Logistic Regression of Vaccination Status in the United States and Finland.

| | The United States | | | Finland | | |
|---|---|---|---|---|---|---|
| | *B* | SE | Odds Ratio | *B* | SE | Odds Ratio |
| Collaboration dimensions | 0.321*** | 0.072 | 1.379 | 0.640*** | 0.140 | 1.897 |
| Social solidarity | 0.035 * | 0.018 | 1.036 | –0.004 | 0.036 | 0.996 |
| Confidence in government | 0.043 | 0.116 | 1.044 | 0.037 | 0.195 | 1.037 |
| Confidence in medicine | 0.505*** | 0.119 | 1.656 | 0.641** | 0.219 | 1.898 |
| Confidence in media | –0.031 | 0.115 | 0.969 | 0.235 | 0.195 | 1.264 |
| Confidence in science | 0.402*** | 0.113 | 1.496 | –0.176 | 0.215 | 0.839 |
| Omnivore media consumer | 0.083 | 0.075 | 1.087 | –0.128 | 0.157 | 0.880 |
| Online hate exposure | 0.383** | 0.131 | 1.467 | 0.105 | 0.220 | 1.110 |
| Male | 0.270* | 0.129 | 1.310 | 0.254 | 0.227 | 1.289 |
| Age | 0.027*** | 0.004 | 1.027 | 0.016** | 0.007 | 1.016 |
| Worry about COVID-19 | 0.083 | 0.099 | 1.086 | 0.336 | 0.199 | 1.399 |
| Ruling party[a] | –0.622*** | 0.142 | 0.537 | 0.545* | 0.230 | 1.725 |
| Constant | –3.23 | 0.495 | 0.039 | –0.917 | 0.960 | 0.400 |

* $p < 0.05$; ** $p < 0.01$; *** $p < 0.001$.
[a]Ruling party is Republican in United States and Liberal Coalition in Finland.

of being vaccinated. Age was positively related to being vaccinated as was identifying as a male. Being exposed to online hate also increased the likelihood of being vaccinated, while Republicans were significantly less likely to be vaccinated. Confidence in the Federal government, confidence in the media, media consumption, and the extent to which you were worried about the pandemic failed to achieve statistical significance in this model.

In Finland, the only significant variables in the model were those previously discussed, and the model performed reasonably well but accounted for less variance than did the American model (–2 log likelihood = 615.49, Naglkerke

## 156   James Hawdon and Donna Sedgwick

$R^2 = 0.195$).[6] As in the United States, believing the relationship between the citizen and the state should be a collaborative partnership increased the odds of being vaccinated. Having confidence in those in charge of the medical institution similarly increased the likelihood of being vaccinated. Age was positively related to being vaccinated. Finally, identifying with one of the political parties that were part of the ruling coalition significantly increased your likelihood of being vaccinated. Members of the ruling party were 73% more likely to be vaccinated than those in the opposition party. No other variables were statistically significant predictors of vaccination status in the Finnish model.

Several important points are evident from these models. First and foremost, it is clear those who view their relationship with their state as a collaborative partnership were far more likely to follow the health-protective recommendation of getting a vaccine once they became available. This supports the findings from Chapter 8 where several of the specific collaborative dimensions predict the intention to be vaccinated. The finding that those dimensions also predict who got vaccinated provides good evidence of the importance of this factor as well as indirect evidence in support of the Theory of Planned Behaviors.

Next, confidence in the medical community and healthcare system were important predictors of vaccination status in both countries. This finding makes intuitive sense given each nation's healthcare system were the ones in charge of providing vaccines. Not having confidence in those who run the system would cause consternation when considering whether to follow their advice. This finding is consistent with previous research among Finns (see Kestilä-Kekkonen et al., 2022). The importance of having confidence in leaders spilled over to the broader scientific community in the United States, but this was not evident in Finland. While exposure to hate was significantly related to vaccination status in the United States, it was not in Finland. This finding could be related to the clear relationship between political party and vaccination status.

As noted above, in both nations, being a member of the more left-leaning party or coalition significantly increased one's odds of being vaccinated. This is unsurprising in Finland since it was the left-leaning party that was recommending vaccinations. In this case, being in the "ruling" instead of the "opposition" party would simply mean that one was complying with the requests of their own party's leadership. However, in the United States, while the government was being run by the more conservative Republican party, it nevertheless recommended vaccinations. In fact, it was the Trump administration that significantly funded *Operation Warp Speed* that supported multiple COVID-19 potential vaccines to speed up their development (US Government Accountability Office, 2021). Although the Trump administration and numerous governmental agencies such as the Center for Disease Control (CDC) encouraged Americans to get vaccinated against the virus, many Republicans refused to follow their own party's advice.

---

[6]Collaborative dimension (odds ratio = 1.88; $p < 0.001$; CI 1.443–2.493); confidence in medical institution (OR = 1.90; $p = 0.003$; CI 1.236–2.916); age (OR = 1.02; $p < 0.035$; CI 1.001–1.031); political party (OR = 1.73; $p = 0.018$; CI 1.099–2.709).

## What Predicts Viewing the State as a Collaborative Partner?

Given the overwhelming evidence that citizens who complied with the health-protective recommendations were those who considered their relationship with the state to be a collaborative one, we need to consider the factors that promote such a perspective. Using the data collected after the pandemic to predict what factors led to adopting a collaborative perspective, we regress our measure of collaboration used in the above logistic regressions on levels of solidarity, if the respondent used multiple media sources, confidence in the federal government and scientific community, if they believed governmental agencies would contribute to ending the pandemic, political party, the extent to which they were worried about COVID-19, age, and sex. Results for both nations are reported in Table 9.2.

Looking at the results, there are striking similarities across the two nations. The models for each nation were statistically significant, and both performed relatively well with the model accounting for 37% of the variation in collaboration in the United States and approximately 32% in Finland. Solidarity, confidence in the federal government, confidence in the scientific community, believing the federal government contributed to ending the pandemic, and being worried about COVID-19 were all significant, positive predictors of viewing one's relationship with their government as being a collaborative partnership. These findings were consistent across nations. Similarly, males were less likely to adopt a collaborative perspective in both the United States and Finland. The relationship between political party and adopting a collaborative perspective was similar in both nations in that members of the left-leaning party or collation were more likely to hold such views and those in the right-leaning party or collation were less likely. Education and confidence in the media were unrelated to holding a collaborative perspective in both nations. Only two cross-national differences emerged in these models. First, being a media omnivore (i.e., consuming multiple forms of news media) was a significant predictor in the United States but not in Finland. In the United States, those who consumed more varied types of media were more likely to believe their relationship with the state should be a collaborative one. Second, age was positively and significantly related to adopting a collaborative perspective in Finland, but this variable failed to achieve significance in the United States.

It is clear from these results the inter-relatedness of the collaborative dimensions with confidence in major institutions and social solidarity. Those who have confidence in social institutions and feel integrated into that system are far more likely to view their relationship with the state in collaborative terms. Given the importance of adopting a collaborative position for predicting who was and who was not vaccinated, and, given the relationship between being vaccinated and becoming ill, these findings highlight the importance of confidence in institutions and trust. As others have noted (e.g., Nocera & McLean, 2023), these are critical factors in how the pandemic was managed and mismanaged. We will discuss this in detail later, but for now, our data provide yet more evidence of the importance of confidence in institutions and solidarity.

Table 9.2. Regression of Collaborative Relationship with the State in the United States and Finland.

| | The United States | | | Finland | | |
|---|---|---|---|---|---|---|
| | $B$ | Standard Error | Standardized Coefficient | $B$ | Standard Error | Standardized Coefficient |
| Solidarity | 0.251*** | 0.024 | 0.224 | 0.215*** | 0.029 | 0.203 |
| Omnivore media consumer | 0.288** | 0.106 | 0.058 | −0.094 | 0.136 | −0.019 |
| Confidence in Federal Government | 0.819*** | 0.155 | 0.132 | .662*** | 0.166 | 0.126 |
| Confidence in Science Community | 1.548*** | 0.141 | 0.253 | 1.247*** | 0.177 | 0.198 |
| Confidence in media | 0.217 | 0.153 | 0.033 | 0.256 | 0.159 | 0.047 |
| Government Helped end pandemic | 0.615*** | 0.096 | 0.148 | 0.746*** | 0.127 | 0.178 |
| Political Party[a] | −0.849*** | 0.203 | −0.090 | 0.393* | 0.188 | 0.056 |
| Worry about COVID-19 | 0.924*** | 0.134 | 0.147 | 1.025*** | 0.162 | 0.170 |
| Age | −0.001 | 0.005 | −0.006 | 0.015* | 0.006 | 0.068 |
| Male | −0.754*** | 0.173 | −0.089 | −0.415* | 0.186 | −0.060 |
| Education | −0.064 | 0.084 | −0.016 | −0.001 | 0.052 | 0.000 |
| Constant | 9.72*** | 0.568 | | 10.37*** | 0.709 | |
| $R^2$ | 0.372 | | | 0.317 | | |

* $p < 0.05$; ** $p < 0.01$; *** $p < 0.001$.
[a]Ruling party is Republican in United States and Liberal Coalition in Finland.

*Pandemic's Effects in Finland and the United States* **159**

It is also clear from our analyses how politics plays out with respect to forming a partnership with one's government. Conservatives in both nations are less likely to view their relationship with the state as a collaborative partnership. While this finding is to be expected given that conservatives are typically more anti-government than are liberals, but it is telling that the relationship between political party and our measure of the collaborative dimensions remains significant even after controlling for other attitudes that should capture traditional conservative hesitancies about the government. That is, while conservatives are more likely to lack confidence in the efficacy of government to solve problems and to hold anti-elite and anti-science attitudes (Atkin, 2017; Mooney, 2007), these factors are controlled for in the equation. As such, the relationship between political party and the collaborative dimensions should be mediated by these other factors; however, despite these factors being the best predictors of collaborative attitudes, they do not mediate the relationship between political party and holding a collaborative perspective.

This finding about collaboration coupled with the importance of political party in predicting who was or was not vaccinated reflects how the pandemic became politicized over time. As the pandemic wore on, one's stance on the pandemic became increasingly related to political affiliation. For example, political party affiliation, but not the political ideologies of liberal and conservative, significantly predicted face mask wearing in the United States (Howard, 2022). Party affiliation was also related to other preventive behaviors, such as social distancing and avoiding public places (e.g., Kiviniemi et al., 2022; Leventhal et al., 2021; Naeim et al., 2021; Pedersen & Favero, 2020; PEW Research Center, 2020). As the pandemic wore on, masking choices, as discussed in Chapter 8, as well as the extent to which one practiced social distancing and their attitudes toward lockdowns, became "a symbol of one's politics" (Nocera & Mclean, 2023, p. 10). We saw this politicization of the pandemic in our data as well, as political party affiliation predicted mask wearing, being vaccinated, and getting boosted. And, as reported in previous chapters, our data provide additional evidence that the politicization of the pandemic became more intense as the pandemic unfolded.

Consequently, the above models lead us to several conclusions. First, being vaccinated and boosted reduced the likelihood of becoming ill with COVID-19. Next, adopting a view that one's relationship with the state should be that of a collaborative partnership, having confidence in central institutions (namely medicine and, in the United States, also science), and social solidarity increased the odds of being vaccinated and boosted, while being politically conservative decreased the odds of being vaccinated and boosted. Finally, having confidence in the government and other major institutions increases the probability that one will believe their relationship with their state is a collaborative one, and being politically conservative decreases that probability. The differences in the overall effects of COVID-19 in the United States and Finland are partially explained by cross-national differences in these factors. Compared to Americans, Finns expressed more confidence in their institutions, were more likely to adopt a collaborative relationship with their state, were more likely to be vaccinated and boosted; and, compared to Americans, COVID-19 was less deadly for Finns than it was for Americans.

## 160  *James Hawdon and Donna Sedgwick*

# A Peek Back

It is now time to consider what we have learned from the previous chapters and the analyses in this chapter. As mentioned above, the plans people made in the early stages of the pandemic mirror what people did. This may not be surprising, but it reaffirms the argument that early perceptions are important and can influence how health crises play out. Let us begin with a peek back.

### Lessons Learned

First, we observed national differences in terms of how people coped with the pandemic, at least in its earliest stages. Americans were significantly more likely to use maladaptive coping strategies and religious coping strategies compared to their Finnish counterparts. Interestingly, however, Americans who used maladaptive strategies in April 2020 did not express significantly lower levels of life satisfaction in November 2020, but Finns who used maladaptive strategies did experience a significant decrease in life satisfaction by November 2020. This again highlights the importance of what behaviors people engage in early in the pandemic can have significant consequences in terms of well-being later in the pandemic. While it appears Americans did not pay a price for using maladaptive strategies, which counters most evidence in the field, the finding also demonstrates how the pandemic dramatically altered our lives. This finding highlights the importance of understanding how powerful major health crises such as the COVID-19 pandemic can alter contexts that then challenge our pre-conceived notions of how the world is supposed to work. We also saw in the current chapter that compliance with the health mandates mattered as people who followed the recommendations were significantly less likely to get sick from COVID-19 multiple times. This finding is yet another piece of evidence that shows the importance of the vaccines in preventing serious illness and developing long-COVID (e.g., Trinh et al., 2024). Given the ravages of long-COVID, it is critically important to avoid contracting the virus multiple times, and our findings suggest following mandates can help reduce the odds of getting sick.

Taken together, the results from these various analyses confirm that what people are thinking and doing in the early stages of a pandemic have long-term consequences. It is therefore important for politicians and public health officials to do everything in their power to persuade people to follow the advice of public health professionals. Yet, these findings also highlight the importance for public health officials and other experts to continue studying how phenomena behave when a crisis significantly alters our experiences and world. We were told throughout the pandemic to "follow the science," and it turns out that much of the science we were told to follow was at least partially correct; however, some of it was not and our confidence in other aspects of "the science" were overstated (see Nocera & Mclean, 2023). We must be humble enough to realize science, and especially any science dealing with humans, is probabilistic and that everything is contextual. Water boils at 100°C under normal conditions, but atmospheric pressure changes that law. Similarly, a health crisis as widespread and serious as COVID-19 changes the context of social relations, and in so doing it has the potential to seriously alter what we think we know about how the world works. It is therefore critical for experts to continue their studies during crises, but they need to do so with a heightened awareness of how the new context ushered in by the crisis may have changed what they thought they understood.

While we believe the above insights are especially important, the most striking and consistent finding from our collective analyses reveals the importance of social solidarity and confidence in our leaders and the institutions they run. We saw these variables play important roles in predicting who was likely to follow various health mandates, and we saw the importance of these factors in influencing respondents' health and well-being. The importance of trust in institutions and fellow citizens should not be surprising. Trust is at the heart of concepts such as social solidarity, social capital, and collective efficacy, and there is an amazingly robust literature linking all these similar concepts to positive social outcomes, be those individual well-being, economic prosperity, crime rates, organizational performance, or community-level health outcomes. Our data and analyses add to this literature. Looking back at our findings, we can see the importance of confidence, trust, and solidarity in terms of being related to coping strategies used to deal with the pandemic, support for spending on various initiatives to combat the pandemic, predicting citizens' commitment to the citizen/state collaborative partnership, compliance with recommendations and mandates, and becoming ill. Indeed, trust in institutions and trust in one's fellow citizens may indeed be the most important variable in determining how well nations, communities, and individuals managed (and survived) the pandemic. As Alan Murray and Nicolas Gordon (2023) say when discussing Joe Nocera and Bethany McLean's *The Big Fail*:

> There's little evidence that countries or communities with hard lockdowns and firm mask mandates did better than those without. There's also little evidence that rich countries did better than poor, or authoritarian societies did better than democratic. In fact, the only variable that seems to explain COVID-19-fighting success is social trust. Societies with relatively high levels of trust – in each other, in their governments, in science, etc. – did better than those without.

Our analyses provide more evidence in support of such assertions, but our findings also speak to what factors influence solidarity and confidence in institutions. For example, we observed that trust in experts strengthened during the initial stages of crisis, but this declined over time. Similarly, satisfaction with the government declined over time, even during the earliest stages of the pandemic. We also saw how media exposure and early ideas about the causes of the pandemic were related to confidence in experts. For example, omnivorous media consumption – or consuming several different forms of media – increased trust in experts as well as satisfaction with the government, but social media-based media consumption was related to the declined trust, especially if this was your

## 162  James Hawdon and Donna Sedgwick

only source of media. We also learned how exposure to online hate materials was influenced by and influenced our levels of confidence in experts and our leaders.

In addition to these insights, we also learned that most people saw the cause of the pandemic as being due to a lack of citizen responsibility and weak restrictive measures on the part of the state, which ultimately is related to trust in our leaders and in each other because this is a function of how people perceive the connection between their social rights and their social obligations. That is, believing the pandemic is due to these factors is a commentary on the individual–state relationship and the belief that the pandemic was a result of both parties failing to live up to their responsibilities. As discussed in several chapters, viewing the relationship between oneself and their government as a collaborative partnership was critically important for predicting compliance, and confidence in institutional leaders and social solidarity increased the chances of viewing the self–state relationship in this manner. But adopting this view is a two-way street: it requires individuals to accept their social responsibilities while simultaneously having the state meet its social obligations.

All of this highlights the importance of maintaining confidence in our leaders, solidarity with our community, and trust in each other during a pandemic. These factors are related to compliance (e.g., Aksoy et al., 2020; Bargain & Aminjonov, 2020; Besley & Dray, 2024; Eichengreen et al., 2021; Marien & Hooghe, 2011; Mishra & Rath, 2020). They are also elements of resilient communities, and resilience is what facilitates managing a crisis as it unfolds and recovering from a crisis after it ends. But our data clearly reveal that our confidence in our leaders and social solidarity waned as the pandemic unfolded, especially among the more conservative among us. As discussed in this chapter and the previous one, the pandemic became politicized, and the partisan divide grew as the pandemic wore on. This is probably the most disturbing part of our findings. Instead of rallying against the threat by pulling together, we resorted to tribalism and turned on each other (Clark & Bain-Selbo, 2022; Lima de Miranda & Snower, 2022).

### Cross-national Differences and Their Implications

We began this chapter by asking the question why Finland fared better than the United States did when it came to COVID-19 outcomes. As discussed in this chapter, part of this difference was due to greater compliance with health mandates, particularly recommendations to vaccinate and get boosted once those options became available. Our data reveal Finns were more likely to do this than were Americans (especially in terms of being boosted). This finding is predictable given Finnish statism compared to the more market-oriented approach found in the United States. Given the importance of confidence in institutions and adopting a collaborative position for predicting vaccination status, we are unsurprised by the finding that Finns complied more and had lower COVID-19-related infection and death rates. Indeed, based on our 2023 data, Finns expressed greater confidence in their leaders than did Americans for every major institution we asked about, which included major companies, the education system, organized religion, the media, the scientific community, the healthcare system, and the major branches

## Pandemic's Effects in Finland and the United States    163

of government. The differences between the countries were all statistically significant.[7] Similarly, Finns expressed significantly more satisfaction with how their federal and local governments handled the pandemic.

While these findings were predicted because of the history of statism and civic cooperation in Finland, it is telling that this relationship was not found in the first two waves of data. In March 2020, Americans expressed significantly more confidence in their institutional leaders than did Finns for banks, major companies, organized religion, the press, the healthcare system, science, and even the executive and legislative branch of government.[8] Thus, at the beginning of the pandemic, the United States had a distinctive advantage over Finland in terms of levels of confidence. However, this advantage began to disappear by November 2020, as the gaps between the two nations closed for every institution, and the difference in confidence in the federal government was no longer statistically significant by then. By the end of the pandemic in 2023, the American advantage in confidence had completely disappeared and the relationship had reversed.

## Conclusion

So, what happened? How did the two nations swap positions regarding the critical variable of confidence in institutional leaders? Well, the short answer is that Finnish leaders and the institutions they ran performed better during the pandemic. As discussed in earlier chapters, Finnish Prime Minister Marin's approach to the pandemic was starkly different than that of US President Trump's. For example, in the earliest days of the pandemic, President Trump downplayed the dangers of the pandemic while Prime Minister Marin noted that, while there was not an epidemic in Finland at the time, the government would remain vigilant. She also relied on her Minister of Social Affairs and Health to reassure the citizens that Finland had good preparedness and masks stockpiled (Koljonen & Palonen, 2021). Thus, the American government's initial response was to deny the dangers of the pandemic. In contrast, the Finnish government's initial response was to alleviate the public's concerns by communicating how the government was acting and providing scientifically informed health information about on the pandemic (Koljonen & Palonen, 2021).

Not only did the initial response of institutional leaders in the two nations differ, the two countries continued to take different approaches. In the United States, numerous mistakes were made. For example, there was frequent tensions between President Trump's office and the nation's leading health advisors about the pandemic – ranging from the importance of testing to the need for masks and other

---

[7]The differences were significant at the $p < 0.001$ level. There was one exception to this. The difference in confidence in major companies was significant at the $p = 0.043$ level, but the direction of the relationship was the same where Finns expressed more confidence than did Americans.

[8]There were no significant differences between the two nations in confidence in the education system.

## 164    James Hawdon and Donna Sedgwick

health-protective behaviors – and these disagreements were frequently reported in the media (see Baker et al., 2020; Haslett, 2020). The obvious inability for the various government agencies to cooperate and coordinate their efforts contributed to the conflicting perspectives and responses between federal and many states' governmental leaders (Subramanian, 2020), as conflicts within governmental agencies can seriously undermine perceptions of competency (see Skidmore, 2016, for a general discussion). In contrast, there was clear and consistent messaging from the Marian administration and her various ministers (Dada et al., 2021; Lindholm et al., 2023; Milne, 2020). As Johan Strang, Associate Professor in Nordic studies at the University of Helsinki said about Prime Minister Marin and other Finnish authorities, "They were calm, in the sense that they can implement quite drastic measures without anybody questioning them" (quoted in Milne, 2020).

In hindsight, the United States made several other mistakes. Their officials implemented widespread lockdowns even in areas where infection rates were low, and they kept these in place for longer than needed. Moreover, their officials overstated the effectiveness of masks and the vaccines. The United States also did not have sufficient stockpiles of equipment, and their general level of preparedness was insufficient (see Nocera & Mclean, 2023). Again, Finland provides a stark contrast. For example, Finland, like Norway and Denmark, imposed a far less severe lockdown than the United States and much of Europe, as most shops and public transportation remained opened. In addition, Finnish law requires it to focus on preparedness, and the preparedness law explicitly mentions pandemics. Thus, the law was triggered at the pandemic's onset, and, unlike the United States and much of the rest of the world, Finland had emergency stockpiles of medical and protective equipment (Milne, 2020). Indeed, compared to the United States, Finland's healthcare infrastructure is far superior for handling a pandemic. For example, based on World Bank data (2024), Finland has 4.3 physicians per 1,000 population while the United States only has 3.6 physicians per 1,000 population. Similarly, the United States has 2.9 hospital beds per 1,000 population while Finland has 3.6 beds per 1,000 population.[9]

In short, compared to the United States (and, indeed, most other nations), Finland was both better prepared for the pandemic and their leaders responded to the crises more effectively. In part because of their preparedness, their leaders were able to reassure the public the nation could manage the crisis, and because of their leaders' responses, the public was more likely to believe them and comply with recommended health-protective behaviors. Consequently, we can and should learn from the Finns how to be better prepared.

---

[9]It is true that the total healthcare expenditures are higher in the United States than in Finland ($12,555 per person compared to $5,599 per person, respectively). However, the United States is very much an outlier, even among high income nations. While Finland is in line with other wealthy nations, the United States spends over three times what would be expected if its healthcare expenditures were in line with other high-income countries. Much of this difference is due to far higher pharmaceutical expenditures.

# References

Abd-Elsalam, S., Noor, R. A., Badawi, R., Khalaf, M., Esmail, E. S., Soliman, S., Abd El Ghafar, M. S., Elbahnasawy, M., Moustafa, E. F., Hassany, S. M. & Medhat, M. A. (2021). Clinical study evaluating the efficacy of ivermectin in COVID-19 treatment: A randomized controlled study. *Journal of Medical Virology*, *93*(10), 5833–5838.

Agrawal, V., Sood, N., & Whaley, C. M. (2023). *The impact of the global COVID-19 vaccination campaign on all-cause mortality* (No. w31812). National Bureau of Economic Research.

Aksoy, C., Eichengreen, B., & Saka, O. (2020). *Young people trust governments less after exposure to an epidemic* [LSE Covid-19 Blog]. https://blogs.lse.ac.uk/covid19/2020/06/22/young-people-trust-governments-less-after-exposure-to-an-epidemic/

Andrejko, K. L. (2022). Effectiveness of face mask or respirator use in indoor public settings for prevention of SARS-CoV-2 infection—California, February–December 2021. *MMWR. Morbidity and Mortality Weekly Report*, *71*.

Arbel, R., & Pliskin, J. (2022). Vaccinations versus lockdowns to prevent COVID-19 mortality. Vaccines, *10*(8), 1347.

Aschhoff, N., & Vogel, R. (2019). Something old, something new, something borrowed: Explaining varieties of professionalism in citizen collaboration through identity theory. *Public Administration*, *97*, 703–720.

Atkeson, A. (2023). *The impact of vaccines and behavior on US cumulative deaths from COVID-19* (No. w31525). National Bureau of Economic Research.

Atkin, E. (2017). *Republicans' war on science just got frighteningly real*. New Republic.

Badman, R. P., Wang, A. X., Skrodzki, M., Cho, H. C., Aguilar-Lleyda, D., Shiono, N., Yoo, S., Chiang, Y., & Akaishi, R. (2022). Trust in institutions, not in political leaders, determines compliance in COVID-19 prevention measures within societies across the globe. *Behavioral Sciences*, *12*(6), 170.

Baker, P., Haberman, M., & Glanz, J. J. (2020). The tensions persist between Trump and medical advisors over the coronavirus. *New York Times* https://www.nytimes.com/2020/04/03/us/politics/coronavirus-trump-medical-advisers.html

Bargain, O., & Aminjonov, U. (2020). Trust and compliance to public health policies in times of COVID-19. *Journal of Public Economics*, *192*, 104316.

Besley, T., & Dray, S. (2024). Trust and state effectiveness: The political economy of compliance. *The Economic Journal*, ueae030.

Bornstein, B. H., & Tomkins, A. J. (Eds.). (2015). *Motivating cooperation and compliance with authority: The role of institutional trust*. Springer International Publishing.

Cerqueti, R., Coppier, R., Girardi, A., & Ventura, M. (2022). The sooner the better: Lives saved by the lockdown during the COVID-19 outbreak. The case of Italy. *The Econometrics Journal*, *25*(1), 46–70.

Chu, D. K., Akl, E. A., Duda, S., Solo, K., Yaacoub, S., Schünemann, H. J., El-Harakeh, A., Bognanni, A., Lotfi, T., Loeb, M. and Hajizadeh, A., (2020). Physical distancing, face masks, and eye protection to prevent person-to-person transmission of SARS-CoV-2 and COVID-19: A systematic review and meta-analysis. *The Lancet*, *395*(10242), pp.1973–1987.

Clark, K. M., & Bain-Selbo, E. (2022). Tribalism and compassion in the age of a pandemic. *Soundings: An Interdisciplinary Journal*, *105*(2), 143–223.

Dada, S., Ashworth, H. C., Bewa, M. J., & Dhatt, R. (2021). Words matter: Political and gender analysis of speeches made by heads of government during the COVID-19 pandemic. *BMJ Global Health*, *6*(1), e003910.

Eichengreen, B., Aksoy, C. G., & Saka, O. (2021). Revenge of the experts: Will COVID-19 renew or diminish public trust in science?. *Journal of Public Economics*, *193*, 104343.

Enright, C., Gilbourne, C., Kiersey, R., Parlour, R., Flanagan, P., McGowan, E., Boland, M., & Mulholland, D. (2024). Efficacy of facemasks in preventing transmission

# 166  James Hawdon and Donna Sedgwick

of COVID-19 in non-healthcare settings: A scoping review. *Journal of Infection Prevention*, 25(1–2), 24–32.

Ford, N., Holmer, H. K., Chou, R., Villeneuve, P. J., Baller, A., Van Kerkhove, M., & Allegranzi, B. (2021). Mask use in community settings in the context of COVID-19: A systematic review of ecological data. *EClinicalMedicine*, 38.

Gupta, S., Cantor, J., Simon, K. I., Bento, A. I., Wing, C., & Whaley, C. M. (2021). Vaccinations against COVID-19 may have averted up to 140,000 deaths in the United States: Study examines role of COVID-19 vaccines and deaths averted in the United States. *Health Affairs*, 40(9), 1465–1472.

Halávka, J. & Rose, A. (2023). The COVID-19 pandemic cost the U.S. economy $14 trillion, new research finds. *Fortune Well*. https://fortune.com/well/2023/05/16/how-much-did-covid-19-pandemic-coronavirus-cost-economy-14-trillion/

Hansen, N. J. H., & Mano, R. C. (2023). Mask mandates save lives. *Journal of Health Economics*, 88, 102721.

Haslett, C. (2020). *Tension with Trump: Dr. Anthony Fouci on telling the truth.* ABCNews. https://abcnews.go.com/Politics/tensions-trump-dr-anthony-fauci-telling-truth/story?id=69750768

Howard, J., Huang, A., Li, Z., Tufekci, Z., Zdimal, V., Van Der Westhuizen, H. M., Von Delft, A., Price, A., Fridman, L., Tang, L. H., & Tang, V. (2021). An evidence review of face masks against COVID-19. *Proceedings of the National Academy of Sciences*, 118(4), p.e2014564118.

Howard, M. C. (2022). Are face masks a partisan issue during the COVID-19 pandemic? Differentiating political ideology and political party affiliation. *International Journal of Psychology*, 57(1), 153–160.

Huang, P. (2021). *How ivermectin became the new focus of the anti-vaccine movement.* NPR. https://www.npr.org/sections/health-shots/2021/09/19/1038369557/ivermectin-anti-vaccine-movement-culture-wars

Jia, K. M., Hanage, W. P., Lipsitch, M., Johnson, A. G., Amin, A. B., Ali, A. R., Scobie, H., & Swerdlow, D. L. (2023). Estimated preventable COVID-19-associated deaths due to non-vaccination in the United States. *European Journal of Epidemiology*, 38(11), 1125–1128.

Juneau, C. E., Briand, A. S., Collazzo, P., Siebert, U., & Pueyo, T. (2023). Effective contact tracing for COVID-19: A systematic review. *Global Epidemiology*, 5, 100103.

Kathi, P. C., & Cooper, T. L. (2005). Democratizing the administrative state: Connecting neighborhood councils and city agencies. *Public Administration Review*, 65(5), 559–567.

Kestilä-Kekkonen, E., Koivula, A., & Tiihonen, A. (2022). When trust is not enough. A longitudinal analysis of political trust and political competence during the first wave of the COVID-19 pandemic in Finland. *European Political Science Review*, 14(3), 424–440.

Kiviniemi, M. T., Orom, H., Hay, J. L., & Waters, E. A. (2022). Prevention is political: Political party affiliation predicts perceived risk and prevention behaviors for COVID-19. *BMC Public Health*, 22(1), 298.

Kluger, J. (2020). Accidental poisonings increased after President Trump's disinfectant comments. *Time*. https://time.com/5835244/accidental-poisonings-trump/

Koljonen, J., & Palonen, E. (2021). Performing COVID-19 CONTROL in Finland: Interpretative topic modelling and discourse theoretical reading of the government communication and hashtag landscape. *Frontiers in Political Science*, 3, 689614.

Lancet. (2023). Long COVID: 3 years in. *Lancet*, 401(10379), 795.

Leventhal, A. M., Dai, H., Barrington-Trimis, J. L., McConnell, R., Unger, J. B., Sussman, S., & Cho, J. (2021). Association of political party affiliation with physical distancing among young adults during the COVID-19 pandemic. *JAMA Internal Medicine*, 181(3), 399–403.

## Pandemic's Effects in Finland and the United States  167

Lima de Miranda, K., & Snower, D. J. (2022). The societal responses to COVID-19: Evidence from the G7 countries. *Proceedings of the National Academy of Sciences, 119*(25), e2117155119.

Lindholm, J., Carlsson, T., Albrecht, F., & Hermansson, H. (2023). Communicating Covid-19 on social media: Analysing the use of Twitter and Instagram by Nordic health authorities and prime ministers. In B. Johansson, Ø. Ihlen, J. Lindholm, & M. Blach-Ørsten (Eds.), *Communicating a pandemic: Crisis management and Covid-19 in the Nordic countries* (pp. 149–172). University of Gothenburg. https://doi.org/10.48335/9789188855688-7

Lyu, W., & Wehby, G. L. (2020). Community use of face masks and COVID-19: Evidence from a natural experiment of state mandates in the US: Study examines impact on COVID-19 growth rates associated with state government mandates requiring face mask use in public. *Health Affairs, 39*(8), 1419–1425.

Marien, S., & Hooghe, M. (2011). Does political trust matter? An empirical investigation into the relation between political trust and support for law compliance. *European Journal of Political Research, 50*(2), 267–291.

Mesle, M. M., Brown, J., Mook, P., Katz, M. A., Hagan, J., Pastore, R., Nitzan, D., Benka, B., Reglberger-Fritz, M., Bossuyt, N., Stouyten, V., Vernemmen, C., Constantinou, E., Maly, M., Kynci, J., Sance, O., Grove Krause, T., Skafte Westergaard, L., … & Pebody, R. (2024). Estimated number of lives directly saved by COVID-19 vaccination programs in the WHO European region, December 2020 to March 2023. *medRxiv,* 2024-01.

Miles, D. K., Stedman, M., & Heald, A. H. (2021). Stay at home, protect the national health service, save lives: A cost benefit analysis of the lockdown in the United Kingdom. *International Journal of Clinical Practice, 75*(3), e13674.

Milne, R. (2020). How Finland kept Covid in check. *Financial Times.* https://www.ft.com/content/61dccfaa-0871-48a2-80ac-dbe6d5b5b5f8

Mishra, C. & Rath, N. (2020). Social solidarity during a pandemic: Through and beyond the Durkheimian Lens. *Social Science & Humanities Open, 2,* 100079.

Mooney, C. (2007). *The Republican war on science.* Hachette UK.

Murray, A., & Gordon, N. (2023). One variable explains why some countries fought COVID better than others—and it's not lockdowns or mask mandates. *Fortune.* https://finance.yahoo.com/news/one-variable-explains-why-countries-053127938.html

Naeim, A., Baxter-King, R., Wenger, N., Stanton, A. L., Sepucha, K., & Vavreck, L. (2021). Effects of age, gender, health status, and political party on COVID-19–related concerns and prevention behaviors: Results of a large, longitudinal cross-sectional survey. *JMIR Public Health and Surveillance, 7*(4), e24277.

Nocera, J., & McLean, B. (2023). *The big fail: What the pandemic revealed about who America protects and who it leaves behind.* Penguin.

Our World in Data. (2024a). *Percent of population at least partially vaccinated.* https://ourworldindata.org/search?q=covid%20

Our World in Data. (2024b). *COVID-19: Contact tracing.* https://ourworldindata.org/search?q=covid%20

Our World in Data. (2024c). *COVID-19: Face covering.* https://ourworldindata.org/search?q=covid%20

Our World in Data. (2024d). *COVID-19: Stringency index.* https://ourworldindata.org/search?q=covid%20

Pedersen, M. J., & Favero, N. (2020). Social distancing during the COVID-19 pandemic: Who are the present and future noncompliers? *Public Administration Review, 80*(5), 805–814.

Pew Research Center. (2020). *Republicans, democrats move even further apart in coronavirus concerns.* https://www.pewresearch.org/politics/2020/06/25/republicans-democrats-move-even-further-apart-in-coronavirus-concerns/

Popp, M., Stegemann, M., Metzendorf, M.I., Gould, S., Kranke, P., Meybohm, P., Skoetz, N., & Weibel, S. (2021). Ivermectin for preventing and treating COVID-19. *Cochrane Database of Systematic Reviews, 7*, 1–159.

Reis, G., Silva, E. A., Silva, D. C., Thabane, L., Milagres, A. C., Ferreira, T. S., dos Santos, V. H. S., Campos, A. M. R., Nogueira, A. P. F. G., de Almeida, E. D., Callegari, A. D. F., Neto, L. C. M., Savassi, M., Simplicio, L. B., Riberio, R., Oliveria, O., Harari, J., Forrest, H., Ruton, S., ..., Mills, E. J. (2022). Effect of early treatment with ivermectin among patients with Covid-19. *New England Journal of Medicine, 386*(18), 1721–1731.

Rivera, J. M., Gupta, S., Ramjee, D., El Hayek, G. Y., El Amiri, N., Desai, A. N., & Majumder, M. S. (2020). Evaluating interest in off-label use of disinfectants for COVID-19. *Lancet Digit Health, 2*(11), e564–e566. https://doi.org/10.1016/S2589-7500(20)30215-6.

Sedgwick, D. (2017). Building collaboration: Examining the relationship between collaborative processes and activities. *Journal of Public Administration Research and Theory, 27*(2), 236–252.

Sedgwick, D., Hawdon, J., Räsänen, P., & Koivula, A. (2022). The role of collaboration in complying with COVID-19 health protective behaviors: A cross-national study. *Administration & Society, 54*(1), 29–56.

Shanka, M. S., & Menebo, M. M. (2022). When and how trust in government leads to compliance with COVID-19 precautionary measures. *Journal of Business Research, 139*, 1275–1283.

Shoukat, A., Vilches, T. N., Moghadas, S. M., Sah, P., Schneider, E. C., Shaff, J., Ternier, A., Chokshi, D., & Galvani, A. P. (2022). Lives saved and hospitalizations averted by COVID-19 vaccination in New York City: A modeling study. *The Lancet Regional Health–Americas, 5*, 1–8.

Skidmore, M. (2016). *Presidents, pandemics, and politics.* Palgrave Macmillan.

Song, Z., Shi, S., & Zhang, Y. (2024). Ivermectin for treatment of COVID-19: A systematic review and meta-analysis. *Heliyon, 10*(6), e27647–e27647.

Spira, B. (2022). Correlation between mask compliance and COVID-19 outcomes in Europe. *Cureus, 14*(4), 1–8.

Subramanian, C. (2020). Governors warn of dire ventilator shortages as virus pandemic rages. Trump says some are playing 'politics'. *USA Today.* https://www.usatoday.com/story/news/politics/2020/04/04/coronavirus-trump-says-states-playing-politics-ventilator-requests/5111963002/.

Thomson, A. M., & Perry, J. L. (2006). Collaboration processes: Inside the black box. *Public Administration Review, 66*(Suppl. 1), 20–32.

Trinh, N. T., Jödicke, A. M., Català, M., Mercadé-Besora, N., Hayati, S., Lupattelli, A., Prieto-Alhambra, D., & Nordeng, H. M. (2024). Effectiveness of COVID-19 vaccines to prevent long COVID: Data from Norway. *The Lancet Respiratory Medicine, 12*, 33–34. https://doi.org/10.1016/S2213-2600(24)00082-1

United States Government Accountability Office. (2021). *Operation warp speed: Accelerated COVID-19 vaccine development status and efforts to address manufacturing challenges.* GOA. https://www.gao.gov/products/gao-21-319

Vigoda, E. (2002). From responsiveness to collaboration: Governance, citizens, and the next generation of public administration. *Public Administration Review, 62*(5), 527–540.

World Bank. (2024). *Physicians per 1,000 people.* https://data.worldbank.org/indicator/SH.MED.PHYS.ZS

Worldometer. (2024). *Coronavirus death toll.* https://www.worldometers.info/coronavirus/coronavirus-death-toll/3/26/2024

Yakusheva, O., van den Broek-Altenburg, E., Brekke, G., & Atherly, A. (2022). Lives saved and lost in the first six months of the US COVID-19 pandemic: A retrospective cost-benefit analysis. *Plos One, 17*(1), e0261759.

Section 4

# A Look Ahead

Chapter 10

# A Look Ahead: How to Better Handle the Next Pandemic and Other Crises

*James Hawdon[a], Donna Sedgwick[a], C. Cozette Comer[a] and Pekka Räsänen[b]*

[a] *Virginia Tech, USA*
[b] *University of Turku, Finland*

### Abstract

The concluding chapter uses insights from the previous chapters to derive recommendations for how to cope with the next pandemic or other crisis. We note the necessity for properly preparing for the next crisis and how such preparation has numerous benefits. Building on the fundamental insight that social solidarity and confidence in those running major institutions was a primary factor in predicting COVID-19 outcomes, we offer a variety of suggestions for building solidarity and confidence prior to the next crisis. Many of these suggestions are related to the dangers of political polarization during crises, and we provide several suggestions for addressing the growing political divide that is evident in many liberal democracies in the early 21st century. We then consider several strategies for maintaining solidarity and confidence during the next crisis. Many of these suggestions focus on how governmental leaders and experts should frame their messages about the crisis and how to best mitigate its effects. Many of these lessons are drawn from the several mistakes that were made during the COVID-19 crisis that have now become visible with hindsight.

*Keywords*: Crisis preparation; social solidarity; message framing; crisis strategy; institutional confidence

---

Perceptions of a Pandemic: A Cross-Continental Comparison of Citizen Perceptions, Attitudes, and Behaviors During COVID-19, 171–182
Copyright © 2025 by James Hawdon, Donna Sedgwick, C. Cozette Comer and Pekka Räsänen
Published under exclusive licence by Emerald Publishing Limited
doi:10.1108/978-1-83608-624-620241010

## 172  *James Hawdon et al.*

## Introduction

The preceding chapters provide insights into what Americans and Finns were thinking and doing in the earliest stages of the COVID-19 pandemic. They also provide insights into what mattered and what seemed to not matter in determining the overall effects of the pandemic. Turning the above findings into prescriptions for the next pandemic is no simple thing, but that is what we aim to do in this closing chapter. There is still much we do not know, and every crisis is different; however, there are some factors that will likely be pertinent regardless of the crisis that confronts us, and we can start there. Our recommendations fall under the umbrella of building trust and confidence in leaders. As seen in earlier chapters and numerous other studies, the role of trust and confidence in leaders and major institutions is critical for ensuring citizens comply with health mandates, and complying with those mandates is vital for successfully managing a crisis. So, how do we build and sustain trust and confidence?

## Building Trust Before the Next Crisis

First, trust and confidence are based on relationships, and we must recognize that it will be hard to build trust in the middle of a pandemic. Given the evidence that political trust tends to erode during pandemics (e.g., Aksoy et al., 2020; Edelman Trust Barometer, 2021; Eichengreen et al., 2021), we need find ways to grow our stock of trust and confidence now so we are better prepared for the next crises. While statist nations like Finland will likely have an easier time building (or re-building) trust and confidence than will more market-oriented, government-wary nations like the United States, it is imperative that nations find ways to build trust and confidence before a crisis brings uncertainty, fear, and inter-group suspicion.

When we consider some factors that are related to trust and confidence, we can draw some conclusions about how to potentially build trust. Doing so will increase our resiliency and can potentially save lives. Failing to do so can have dire consequences. As Cevat Giray Aksoy et al. (2020, p. 7) say:

> One can envisage a scenario where low levels of trust allow an epidemic to spread, and where the spread of the epidemic reduces trust in government still further, hindering the ability of the authorities to contain future epidemics and address other social problems.

We therefore offer the following six recommendations for building trust and confidence in institutions *prior to* the next crisis.

- First, political divides erode trust and confidence in institutions. It is difficult to build trust during a time when political parties are determined to "win at all costs" and never concede a victory to the other side. We must therefore address the growing political divide, which is particularly stark in the two-party United

States, but also in many European countries, including Finland (Koivula et al., 2021). It should be noted that while political polarization has been growing and becoming more divisive over the years, there are sizable portions of the public that agree on many fundamental issues. These areas of agreement must be acknowledged and used to build bridges. To do this, we need to recognize that we agree on most goals. While we may differ on the means to achieve these, that is the essence of democracy. Working those differences out is the art of compromise, and it is possible to do that with open, constructive dialogue where our political opponents are seen as people who disagree instead of mortal enemies (see Hawdon, 2024).

- Second, political divides are amplified by misinformation and filter bubbles. Misinformation and disinformation fuel fear and division, especially when these are amplified in echo-chambers or online filter bubbles. Because social media is driven by personalizing algorithms that feed users information and advertisements based on their previous browsing history, like-minded people are sorted into various bubbles (see Pariser, 2011, for a detailed discussion). We know that tight cliques that are not well connected to other cliques impede the flow of information (see Granovetter, 1983), which in turn leads to people becoming more rigid in their thinking. These online filter bubbles help drive political polarization (Hawdon, 2024). Basically, when we see evidence that supports our bubble's views, we often assume our view is correct without considering evidence from other positions or the other side; and, personalized algorithms make it amazingly easy to find "evidence" in support of one's view. This creation of echo-chambers of unverified claims fuel conspiracies, and these can pose dangerous barriers to people accessing and using personal health information (see Holone, 2016). While it is unlikely that tech companies are going to stop using personalizing algorithms or that governments will intervene and outlaw these, governments could step-up and at the least provide the public more information about the use of these algorithms and their effects. Humans have sorted themselves into groups of like-minded people for a long time; but, prior to online personalizing algorithms, we were aware that we were self-sorting and that others held different opinions. We need to be equally aware that this is happening online to avoid the most dangerous consequences of filter bubbles.
- Third, it is not only online filter bubbles that divide us. Other forms of media are also contributing to the division. As reported in the chapter on media consumption and confidence in institutional leaders, omnivore media consumers who consumed multiple sources of media were more likely to express high levels of trust. Like busting online filter bubbles, busting media bubbles would facilitate information dissemination and expose people to differing opinions and perspectives. There is no straightforward way to bust these media filter bubbles, but media companies could be required to better represent multiple perspectives. The *Fairness Doctrine*, which was policy formulated by the US Federal Communications Commission and regulated licensed broadcasters in the United States from 1949 to 1987, required fair and balanced coverage of controversial issues of interest and mandated networks devote time to

174 *James Hawdon et al.*

contrasting views on issues of public importance. While there were problems with the *Fairness Doctrine*, it did prevent license broadcasters from presenting overly biased perspectives and questionably factual information. Revisiting such legislation should at least be considered.

- Fourth, and related to the above points, we desperately need better education on data literacy. A study by Matthew Mettler and Jeffery Mondak (2024) asked 2,000 adults to say if 12 statements were fact or opinion. Disturbingly, the researchers found that fewer than 5% of adults could correctly identify all 12 statements. These findings raise serious concerns about our abilities to engage in effective dialogue. After all, it will be extremely difficult to agree on what to do about some particular fact when we cannot even agree on what the facts are. While these findings were based on a sample of Americans, we suspect the finding is applicable, at least to some degree, in other nations because of lapses in data literacy. The 24/7 news cycle has not helped with our data literacy as programs include lengthy discussions of opinions by "experts." Rarely, if ever, do these "experts" acknowledge when they move from reporting the facts to interpreting them and espousing their opinion about the fact. Thus, in the short term, policies such as a revised *Fairness Doctrine* could at least require broadcasters to clearly label their programming as "factual" or "editorial." Ultimately, however, the responsibility falls on the citizenry to be informed. Consequently, in the long term, we need to improve our data-literacy education so people can develop their critical thinking skills to differentiate fact from opinion.
- Fifth, we need to recognize an additional role that "experts" play in the trust and confidence equation: namely, we trust those who have proven themselves to be competent. We saw in the earlier chapters that trust and confidence in institutional leaders increased in the initial stages of the pandemic in Finland, but it decreased in the United States. This is undoubtedly partially due to Finland's better preparedness to deal with the pandemic. To prepare for the next health crisis, nations need to follow Finland's lead. At the very least, nations should (1) stockpile Personal Protective Equipment (PPE), (2) develop and reinforce alternative PPE supply chains, (3) design, review, and evaluate a national contact tracing strategy, and (4) develop protocols for better protecting the most vulnerable (i.e., the elderly, those with comorbidities) who were disproportionately affected by COVID-19 and likely would be by any disease. Being better prepared would allow our medical experts and politicians to manage the crisis more effectively, which, in turn, would increase the public's confidence in them.
- Finally, and related to the last point, it is simply a fact that even the most learned among us does not know everything. Science, especially any science of humans, is probabilistic. It is also a simple fact that scientists make mistakes. While we ultimately want our "experts" to be right, people can tolerate them being wrong if they do not believe they were misled. Joel Vos (2021) calls for the need for what he calls the "World Resilience Society." In this society, scientists and governmental spokespersons acknowledge risk and uncertainties. By this he means,

*A Look Ahead* **175**

> Throughout their decisions and communications, scientists and governments mention the risks, variations and uncertainties involved; their communication is transparent and facilitates critical public debate. If they present any symbols or imaginings … they are explicit about their ontological status: this is our vision, not Reality. (Vos, 2021, p. 146)

The formation of such a society and such an approach to knowledge would be refreshing and would go a long way toward reinstalling trust and confidence in our leaders and experts.

These six steps can help restore the confidence we have in our leaders and institutions. Doing so can help us not only potentially slow the crises, but it can also help us solve it. To be sure, building trust and confidence in our institutions will not be easy, but it very well might make the difference between a crisis and a devastating crisis.

## Sustaining Trust During a Crisis

While it is critically important for nations to build (or rebuild) levels of trust and confidence in their institutions prior to the next crisis, another crisis is inevitable. It is not a matter of if, but when. Climate change, further human encroachment into wildlife habitats, and the shrinking of the human world through globalization will undoubtedly unleash new crises that upend our lives and threaten our very existence. Being prepared helps, but we will also have to respond as the crisis unfolds before us. As we saw in the previous chapters, how we respond will likely vary. Moreover, how we respond will likely influence the overall effects of the crisis. So, we now turn to what can be done *during the crisis* to help mitigate its effects.

The previous chapters provided much information concerning the importance of people viewing their relationship with the state as a collaborative partnership. Much of this is about their perceptions of solidarity with each other and trust and confidence in those leading their nation's major institutions. As just discussed, this confidence can be dramatically influenced by how leaders and experts perform during the crisis. Specifically, this confidence will be related to how they frame their messages about the crisis. The basic goal of those politicians and other leaders in issuing messages is to convince the population to behave in a specific way (i.e., follow their advice about health protective behaviors), and to do this they must convince people that their behaviors will be rewarding (or at least allow them to avoid a punishment such as becoming ill or dying). As we know from basic behavioral psychology, a behavior will likely occur if the rewards of the behavior are perceived to outweigh the punishments of the behavior. It may seem like it would be easy enough to frame health protective behaviors as being more rewarding than punishing, especially when you are discussing a deadly disease; however, there are critical pitfalls that politicians, healthcare providers, scientific experts, and other institutional leaders must avoid if they are to maintain the levels of public confidence needed to induce compliance.

**176** *James Hawdon et al.*

Given the importance of trust and confidence in the leaders of major institutions for bringing about compliance with health protective behaviors, any messaging about the pandemic from politicians, experts, and other leaders needs to be carefully crafted to promote confidence. Drawing on a large literature dedicated to the study of effective health communication (e.g., Berry, 2006; Coulter et al., 1998; Kahan, 2010; Witte, 1995), we can make the following suggestions about how to frame messages about crises in general and health crises in particular.

- First, any effective messaging must make its claim in a clear and understandable manner. Research shows that the general public's reading and comprehensive skills in the United States and Finland are relatively high (see NCES, 2024); nevertheless, medical issues can be complex and filled with uncertainties. These conditions complicate issuing straightforward, understandable messaging. Nevertheless, healthcare providers need to distill the threat's basics and present them in a way that most of their public understands. The message should emphasize the personal health risks while highlighting the collective health consequences associated with not following health mandates (Berry, 2006; Coulter et al., 1998; Kim & Kreps, 2020; Motta et al., 2021; Witte, 1995). These are fundamental aspects of the collaborative relationship that are so important for compliance (see Sedgwick et al., 2022; Chapter 9 of this volume), and they should be front-and-center in any messaging about the crisis. While there is evidence that a fear-based approach is effective at motivating compliance, the information about the risks associated with non-compliance needs to be honest and should avoid being alarmist (Coulter et al., 1998). A message that "everybody is going to die" is quickly refuted when one person survives, and one piece of counterevidence can effectively undermine the trust the public has in those officials issuing the claims. Thus, the message must strike a balance between highlighting the risks without overstating them. In addition, the message must strike the balance between being readily understandable without using patronizing language. Framing messages in this way can even overcome strong partisan divides (see Motta et al., 2021).
- Second, the messaging must be consistent. Consistent messaging allows people to better understand the risks of non-compliance and benefits of compliance. This would make it easier to remember the message and the advice it contains. It will also help build trust, provided the message is accurate. While the importance of consistent messaging is clear, many governments unfortunately failed to provide it about COVID-19. For example, while most Asian governments mandated wearing face coverings in public from the very beginning of the pandemic, most Western governments, including both the United States and Finland, did not recommend wearing masks at first. Many governments, such as the US government, recommended not wearing masks due to PPE shortages to ensure medical staff had a sufficient supply. Indeed, most Western nations did not recommend mask-wearing until they faced dramatic increases in the numbers of infected people. This inconsistent messaging undoubtedly fostered confusion, led to people questioning the efficacy of masks, and heightened mistrust toward health professionals (e.g., Zhang et al., 2021). A more consistent

message about masks could have led to greater compliance with the request to wear them. To be sure, the messages we give at the beginning of a crisis may need to alter as the crisis unfolds. The COVID-19 pandemic exposed us to a new virus that we knew almost nothing about. No one really was sure what to do as this was truly an unprecedented event. Recognizing this, it may be necessary to change the messaging; however, when such changes are needed, they must be clearly explained and justified. Failure to explain and justify the changes in messaging will surely undermine the confidence people have in their leaders.

- Third, the importance of consistency in messaging not only applies to messaging over time, but it also applies to messaging between actors. That is, the messaging must not only stay the same as the pandemic progresses but also be consistent regardless of who is giving it. Here we saw stark differences between the United States and Finland. As discussed in Chapter 6, the rhetoric used by President Trump and Prime Minster Marian were quite different, and while President Trump actively questioned or refuted what experts said (see, e.g., Poznanski, 2020), Prime Minister Marian typically let her Minsters and science experts do the talking. It is unsurprising to us then that confidence in leaders increased in Finland but decreased in the United States as the pandemic unfolded.

- Fourth, the message must be believable. This aspect of messaging may very well be the most important. One can always provide clarifying information to make a message more believable and justify any inconsistencies in messaging, but once the message's believability is lost, it is extremely difficult to regain it. As noted above, it can be easy to falsify claims if they are exaggerated. For example, many governmental leaders misled the public by intentionally downplaying the seriousness of the pandemic. For example, President Trump repeatedly claimed that the virus would "just go away," claiming it would do so by April 2020 (see Wolfe & Dale, 2020). Similarly, it was a mistake to claim that the vaccines would prevent one from becoming infected with COVID-19 or spreading it since the evidence never suggested they would. What the evidence suggested – and still shows – is that the vaccines reduced the likelihood of infection and, most importantly, the likelihood of severe illness. Yet, this did not stop officials from claiming otherwise. For example, Center for Disease Control (CDC) Director Rochelle Walensky clearly overstated the case when she said on national television that, "Our data from the CDC today suggest that vaccinated people do not carry the virus, don't get sick, and that it's not just in the clinical trials but it's also in real-world data." Similarly, Chief Medical Advisor to the President Anthony Fauci told the *Face the Nation* audience that, in those who may become infected "the level of virus is so low, it makes it extremely unlikely … they will transmit it" (quoted in Nocera & McLean, 2023, pp. 309–310). Thus, the vaccines undoubtedly achieved their most important goal of preventing most hospitalizations and deaths from COVID-19, and they did this without widespread serious side effects, but the experts clearly overstated their effectiveness in preventing illness (see Nocera & McLean, 2023). While it is understandable that health experts and politicians want to

## 178    *James Hawdon et al.*

hype a "silver bullet" type solution to an ongoing crisis – especially when there is evidence that the "silver bullet" will help as there was with the vaccines – it is unwise to overpromise. Once again, it takes only one vaccinated person becoming ill with the disease to call into question experts who claimed that would not happen, and as such "breakthrough infections" mounted, confidence in the experts waned. Research indicates that honestly expressing uncertainty increases institutional trust (e.g., Badman et al., 2022), and politicians and experts will be wise to acknowledge they do not have all the answers, their solutions are based on the "best available data," and it is unlikely that any one solution will be completely effective for everyone under all circumstances. This was the tactic taken by Prime Minister Marin's administration when they provided scientifically informed health information about the pandemic (see Koljonen & Palonen, 2021; Lindholm et al., 2023). Scientific research can teach us a lot, but there is always uncertainty in our understanding. Contrary to what politicians and experts may think, admitting that can promote trust rather than undermine it. Humility goes a long way in building trusting relationships. Although the exact approach should be tailored to the context (e.g., audience, types of uncertainty), clearly and consistently communicating uncertainty in science can build trust and confidence (Gustafson & Rice, 2020).

- Fifth, the message must not only be understandable, consistent, and believable, it must be accurate and complete (Kim & Kreps, 2020). While understating the threats and/or over-promising the solutions can undermine trust and confidence, so can providing incomplete information. For example, several information deficits pertaining to masks have been identified. As previously mentioned, the scientific efficacy of mask wearing was not fully discussed and revealed, but other deficits also shaped the mask debate. There was incomplete information about the safe use of masks, how to properly clean them or reuse them, and how to safely dispose of them (Zhang et al., 2021). A similar story can be told about the attempt to find other therapeutic cures or preventatives such as the various antiviral drugs that were tried on or specifically developed for COVID-19.
- Sixth, the counter-messaging that aims to undermine the position of experts must be aggressively addressed. Institutional leaders need to realize there will always be those offering opposing opinions, so they must establish information diffusion strategies that afford them control over the contents of the message to eliminate confusion (Kim & Kreps, 2020). Doing this will not be easy, however. As Hardey (1999) observed years ago, the Internet provides a forum through which the hierarchical model of information giving is challenged, and with this challenge comes a shift in power in the doctor–patient relationship. Those who already distrust scientific experts tend to be particularly resistant to expert messaging (Merkley, 2020), and anti-science attitudes were barriers to expert-sourced messaging about the COVID-19 vaccine (Cohen, 2020). Experts need to realize that these narratives will exist, and they must find a way to both learn from them as well as counter them. Of course, countering oppositional narratives can be particularly difficult in modern liberal democracies where there is a tremendous amount of diverse information. The openness and unrestricted press and Internet found in liberal democracies make controlling any narrative nearly

impossible, especially with the growth of non-traditional media sources and social networking sites. While the diverse information sources found in liberal democracies deliver more information to individuals, and this information can allow for greater consideration of the data, it often causes the spread of incorrect and biased information. It also contributes to selective information processing and sharing among people, especially during times of heightened polarization, because we tend to accept what reinforces our own beliefs but also what supports our tribe (see Clark & Bain-Selbo, 2022). It is therefore critical that governments and experts provide access to credible public health organizations to avoid information overload (see Goto et al., 2014; Kim & Kreps, 2020). The World Health Organization (WHO) offered such sources, but it was likely too late by the time they did. Confidence in WHO had already been depleted. Trust and confidence in institutions erodes more during pandemics and crises in democracies than it does in autocracies (see Aksoy et al., 2020; also see Edelman Trust Barometer, 2021), in large part because democratic regimes find consistent messaging more difficult. Consequently, liberal democracies need to act very quickly to create, publicize, and provide access to these sources.

- Seventh, we must carefully address fundamental tensions between the above recommendations. There is inherent tension between keeping a message simple while simultaneously making it accurate and complete. There is also a fundamental tension between convincing people of the necessity of them complying with recommendations and not over promising on what benefits compliance will confer and risks it will avoid. There is also a tension between having a consistent message over time and keeping the message accurate as new information is gathered, processed, and analyzed. These tensions are always present and cannot be avoided; however, effective communicators should consider these tensions and craft messages that balance them. We do not offer a strategy for doing this, but we do advise that those trying to craft messages be aware of these tensions and thoughtfully consider how they are to be managed.
- Finally, experts and politicians must be aware that there are many who do not trust them (Cohen, 2020; Merkley, 2020), and that science has been under attack from various groups – including some mainstream groups – for some time (see, e.g., Atkin, 2017). As such, there will always be skeptics, and this becomes especially true in hyper-polarized environments like those that exist in most democracies today. In hyper-politicized environments, political opponents often want to deny the other side a "win," even if doing so is clearly not in the best interest of the nation. We saw this during the pandemic as mask wearing and the vaccines became politicized in both nations we studied. These health protective behaviors became symbols of one's political tribe, and the anti-mask and anti-vax tribe was quick to publicize their skepticism about the health measures their governments and the expert agencies such as the WHO were promoting. While some of this skepticism was undoubtedly due to political tribalism, ignorance, and irrationality, some of it was not. After all, some skepticism – about everything – is healthy. Some disagreement is not due to ignorance, a misunderstanding of the facts, or contempt for one's political rival; some disagreement is due to differences in interpretation of facts and/or differing priorities. We can understand

## 180  *James Hawdon et al.*

these differences in terms of what Haidt (2012; also see Iyer et al., 2012) calls "moral foundations." Specifically in terms of a health crisis like the COVID-19 pandemic, several of Haidt's moral foundations were evident in the fights over health recommendations. Clearly, people emphasized "care" as people wanted to save others' lives and protect us from the virus's harms. But there were also the moral foundations of "fairness" and "liberty." Yes, everyone wanted to care for others and protect them from harm, but should this burden be distributed equally or proportionately? That is, was it fair to shut down the economy and demand people stay at home when doing so was far less costly to those who could work remotely in comfortable private homes with large yards than it was to those who lost their jobs and were forced to stay in their three-room apartment? Should this burden been distributed more equably, or should the burden have only fallen on those living in areas with high rates of infection? Should the government have limited everyone's freedom when it became clear early in the pandemic that certain people (i.e., the elderly and those with underlying health conditions) were far more at risk than were the young? Should they have paid the price of widespread shutdowns when their risk levels were relatively low? We are not advocating which moral foundation should be maximized. The point is that these positions exist, and the ones people emphasize have a lot to do with their perspective and if they believe the messaging of politicians and experts. Given that these differing positions exist, those crafting the message need to be aware of them and not to simply dismiss those who disagree with them as being "irrational" or "selfish" or "overly righteous." There are ways to craft a message to persuade those who disagree with you, and politicians and experts would be wise to learn these tactics. For example, research suggests that messages are more likely to persuade skeptics if they recognize and validate the skeptics' concerns (Kahan, 2010) and discuss alternative positions openly and honestly (Coulter et al., 1998). If we are cognizant that rational people can honestly disagree over alternative courses of actions and avoid dismissing them and their ideas, we are likely to not only craft more effective messages but also develop more trusting relationships and perhaps restore our confidence in our institutional leaders. Doing this needs to be the goal because, as we saw in the previous pages, it matters a lot.

## Conclusion

The chapters in this book demonstrate differences in how people and their governments responded to the COVID-19 pandemic. As we document, these early responses had both immediate and long-lasting consequences. We chose to compare the United States and Finland because, while both wealthy liberal democracies with well-developed healthcare systems, they provided a stark contrast in approaches to governance and social welfare. The comparison between these nations provided insights concerning what each citizenry considered to be important and what behaviors they each chose to perform. The observed cross-national differences provided insights into policies and strategies that were and were not overly effective. Based on these insights, we offer the above recommendations.

## A Look Ahead    *181*

While following these recommendations may not prevent the next pandemic or other crisis, they should help keep it from becoming as politicized as the COVID-19 pandemic did. If that can be achieved and societies can maintain their levels of trust and confidence in their leaders and the experts best trained to deal with the specifics of the crisis, it is highly likely the crisis's ill effects will be mitigated. Doing so will not be easy, but it will be well worth the effort.

## References

Aksoy, C., Eichengreen, B., & Saka, O. (2020). *Young people trust governments less after exposure to an epidemic*. LSE Covid 19 Blog.

Atkin, E. (2017). *Republicans' war on science just got frighteningly real*. New Republic.

Badman, R. P., Wang, A. X., Skrodzki, M., Cho, H. C., Aguilar-Lleyda, D., Shiono, N., Yoo, S., Chiang Y., & Akaishi, R. (2022). Trust in institutions, not in political leaders, determines compliance in COVID-19 prevention measures within societies across the globe. *Behavioral Sciences, 12*(6), 170.

Berry, D. (2006). *Health communication: Theory and practice*. McGraw-Hill Education (UK).

Clark, K. M., & Bain-Selbo, E. (2022). Tribalism and compassion in the age of a pandemic. *Soundings: An Interdisciplinary Journal, 105*(2), 143–223.

Cohen, E. (2020). *Fauci says Covid-19 vaccine may not get U.S. to herd immunity if too many people refuse to get it*. https://www.cnn.com/2020/06/28/health/fauci-coronavirus-vaccine-contact-tracing-aspen/index.html

Coulter, A., Entwistle, V., & Gilbert, D. (1998). *Informing patients: An assessment of the quality of patient information materials*. King's Fund.

Edelman Trust Barometer. (2021). *Global report*. https://www.edelman.com/sites/g/files/aatuss191/files/2022-01/2022%20Edelman%20Trust%20Barometer_FullReport.pdf

Eichengreen, B., Aksoy, C. G., & Saka, O. (2021). Revenge of the experts: Will COVID-19 renew or diminish public trust in science?. *Journal of Public Economics, 193*, 104343.

Goto, A., Rudd, R. E., Lai, A. Y., Yoshida, K., Suzuki, Y., Halstead, D. D., Yoshid-Komiya, H., & Reich, M. R. (2014). Leveraging public health nurses for disaster risk communication in Fukushima City: A qualitative analysis of nurses' written records of parenting counseling and peer discussions. *BMC Health Services Research, 14*, 1–9.

Granovetter, Ma. (1983). The strength of weak ties: A network theory revisited. *Sociological Theory, 1*(1), 201–233.

Gustafson, A., & Rice, R. E. (2020). A review of the effects of uncertainty in public science communication. *Public Understanding of Science, 29*(6), 614–633. https://doi.org/10.1177/0963662520942122

Haidt, J. (2012). *The righteous mind: Why good people are divided by politics and religion*. Vintage.

Hardey, M. (1999). Doctor in the house: The Internet as a source of lay health knowledge and the challenge to expertise. *Sociology of Health & Illness, 21*, 820–835.

Hawdon, J. (2024, March 19). *Political violence and extremism* [Paper presentation]. CHI St. Joseph children's health ending violence in our community conference, Lancaster, Pennsylvania.

Holone, H. (2016). The filter bubble and its effect on online personal health information. *Croatian Medical Journal, 57*(3), 298.

Iyer, R., Koleva, S., Graham, J., Ditto, P., & Haidt, J. (2012). Understanding libertarian morality: The psychological dispositions of self-identified libertarians. *PLOS One*, 1–23. https://journals.plos.org/plosone/article?id=10.1371/journal.pone.0042366

Kahan, D. (2010). Fixing the communications failure. *Nature, 463*(7279), 296–297.

## 182  James Hawdon et al.

Kim, D. K. D., & Kreps, G. L. (2020). An analysis of government communication in the United States during the COVID-19 pandemic: Recommendations for effective government health risk communication. *World Medical & Health Policy*, *12*(4), 398–412.

Koivula, A., Räsänen, P., Oksanen, A., & Keipi, T. (2021). Risk response over time: Political compartmentalization of terrorism risk perception. *Journal of Risk Research*, *24*(7), 781–795.

Koljonen, J., & Palonen, E. (2021). Performing COVID-19 control in Finland: Interpretative topic modelling and discourse theoretical reading of the government communication and hashtag landscape. *Frontiers in Political Science*, *3*, 689614.

Lindholm, J., Carlsson, T., Albrecht, F., & Hermansson, H. (2023). Communicating Covid-19 on social media: Analysing the use of Twitter and Instagram by Nordic health authorities and prime ministers. In B. Johansson, Ø. Ihlen, J. Lindholm, & M. Blach-Ørsten (Eds.), *Communicating a pandemic: Crisis management and Covid-19 in the Nordic countries* (pp. 149–172). University of Gothenburg. https://doi.org/10.48335/9789188855688-7

Merkley, E. (2020). Anti-intellectualism, populism, and motivated resistance to expert consensus. *Public Opinion Quarterly*, *84*(1), 24–48. https://doi.org/10.1093/poq/nfz053

Mettler, M., & Mondak, J. J. (2024). *Fact-opinion differentiation*. Harvard Kennedy School Misinformation Review. https://misinforeview.hks.harvard.edu/article/fact-opinion-differentiation/

Motta, M., Sylvester, S., Callaghan, T., & Lunz-Trujillo, K. (2021). Encouraging COVID-19 vaccine uptake through effective health communication. *Frontiers in Political Science*, *3*, 630133.

National Center for Educational Statistics (NCES). (2024). Program for International Student Assessment *(PISA) Reading Literacy results*. PISA 2022 U.S. Results – Reading Literacy – International Comparisons of Student Achievement (ed.gov).

Nocera, J., & McLean, B. (2023). *The big fail: What the pandemic revealed about who America protects and who it leaves behind*. Penguin.

Pariser, E. (2011). *The filter bubble: How the new personalized web is changing what we read and how we think*. Penguin.

Poznanski, M. (2020). Apparently Trump ignored early coronavirus warnings that has consequences. *The Washington Post*. https://www.washingtonpost.com/politics/2020/03/23/apparently-trump-ignored-early-coronavirus-warnings-that-has-consequences/

Sedgwick, D., Hawdon, J., Räsänen, P., & Koivula, A. (2022). The role of collaboration in complying with COVID-19 health protective behaviors: A cross-national study. *Administration & Society*, *54*(1), 29–56.

Vos, J. (2021). *The psychology of COVID-19: Building resilience for future pandemics*. SAGE.

Witte, K. (1995). Fishing for success: Using the persuasive health message framework to generate effective health campaigns. In E. Maibach & R. L. Parrott (Eds.), *Designing health messages: Approaches from communication theory and public health practice* (pp. 145–156). Sage.

Wolfe, D., & Dale, D. (2020). *It's going to disappear: A timeline of Trump's claims that Covid-19 will vanish*. CNN. https://www.cnn.com/interactive/2020/10/politics/covid-disappearing-trump-comment-tracker/

Zhang, Y. S. D., Young Leslie, H., Sharafaddin-Zadeh, Y., Noels, K., & Lou, N. M. (2021). Public health messages about face masks early in the COVID-19 pandemic: Perceptions of and impacts on Canadians. *Journal of Community Health*, *46*(5), 903–912.

# Methodological Appendix

## Data Collection Procedure and Description of Variables Used

### Data Description

The book utilizes survey data collected in April and November 2020. In addition, in the final chapter we also use a similar data set that was collected in November 2023, approximately 6 months after the pandemic was officially declared over. The Economic Sociology Unit at the University of Turku, Finland, and the Center for Peace Studies and Violence Prevention at Virginia Tech, United States, were responsible for data collection procedures for each round.

Unlike many other surveys conducted in 2020, our surveys included many of the same people in both the first and second waves. This book is based on data that have a panel of respondents from two countries. The unique longitudinal data generated from these surveys permit us to assess the effects of COVID-19 within and between individuals and countries. While our third wave of data is a separate sample and not panel data, we gathered data that tap similar concepts that were used in the first two waves of data and then correlate these with health and well-being outcomes related to the pandemic.

This Appendix serves as a technical chapter that describes the data in detail. It also includes detailed descriptions of how all the concepts used in the analyses throughout the book are measured. Here, you will find a summary of data collection procedure and description of the variables used in the content chapters without the distraction of the methodological and statistical details.

### Data Collection Procedure

The first round of surveys was collected in April 2020, and the second in November 2020. Of these two surveys, panel survey data were created consisting of the respondents who answered in both rounds 1 and 2. An additional third round of surveys was collected in November 2023. Random samples of Finnish and American residents were invited to participate in online surveys administrated by Dynata company, which is a global provider of data solutions and technology for consumer and business-to-business survey research. Each respondent came from demographically balanced samples, which were based on quota estimations by the data provider (Dynata, 2024). The targeted population were 16–76-year-old Finns and Americans.

In the first round, there were a total of 3,000 respondents (1,500 from both Finland and the United States) and 3,108 respondents in the second (1,537 from Finland and 1,535 from the United States). Out of the original 3,000 respondents,

## 184 *Methodological Appendix*

767 respondents from Finland and 613 respondents from the United States answered both the first and second rounds of the survey forming the panel data. Therefore, the panel data consist of 1,380 respondents. These second wave of data also includes 733 new Finnish respondents and 887 new American respondents, so the total sample size for wave 2 was also 1,500 for both nations.

An additional third round of surveys was collected using a similar online survey and was also administrated by Dynata. Unlike in the 2020 samples, however, all respondents were new recruits who had not participated in the study earlier. The final sample size was 3,177, out of which 1,599 were Finnish respondents and 1,578 were Americans. The questionnaire in the third round included some items that were the same as in the first two waves; however, it also included new items that were relevant for understanding more recent changes in the aftermath of COVID-19 pandemic. The latest data are primarily used in chapter nine of the book.

Pre-recruited panel surveys are nonprobability samples; however, nonprobability proportional sampling panels are demographically balanced on important population characteristics. Comparing our samples to census figures from both nations reveal that the samples are reflective of the population in terms of sex within the expected margin of error. They are also generally reflective of the population with respect to age, although middle-aged people 45–64 are slightly over-represented and older people aged 65 or over are underrepresented in Finland. These departures from the overall population were relatively minor and did not significantly alter the substantive findings. Therefore, the samples reasonably reflect the general populations. Importantly, evidence suggests that probability and nonprobability samples yield similar results when using online surveying platforms (Parti et al., forthcoming; Simmons & Bobo, 2015; Weinberg et al., 2014).

## Measurement and Description of General Background Variables

Comparative data analyses presented in this book are conducted utilizing data sets originating from two distinct national contexts, Finland and the United States. Given the differences in the socio-political landscapes and institutional frameworks of these nations, it becomes necessary to ensure the comparability of survey metrics employed in the study. To address this, the survey was originally constructed in English and then translated into Finnish by three members of the research team who are native Finnish speakers and fluent in English. The survey was then re-translated into English to provide a quality check for comparability. In addition, our methodological approach included modification of numerous variables within the original data sets. This procedural adjustment was essential to facilitate the cross-national comparison and ensure the validity of the comparative analysis.

The primary motivation of our study is to compare perceptions and experiences between the two nations. As all the surveys targeted residents of Finland or the United States, the respondent's nationality was taken simply from data status

*Methodological Appendix* **185**

information. We describe the measurement and re-coding procedures of our general background variables below.

First, information on respondent's *age* is crucial in all sociological analysis. Age was measured with question: "How old were you on your last birthday," which provides current age in years. In the analyses throughout the book, age is used as continuous variable. Certain chapters also use age as a categorical variable so that that it captures different life-phases. For this purpose, the categorized five are groups are 16–24-year-olds, 25–34-year-olds, 35–44-year-olds, 45–54-year-olds, and 55–67-years-olds.

Similarly, *sex* is one of the key background variables usually included in survey studies. Sex was measured using question: "Are you ..." with options to choose from being either "male," female" or "other." Option "other" were recorded as system missing because each of the samples included only one to five respondents choosing this option (less than 0.05% of individuals participating in the study). In other words, sex is treated in the analysis as a dichotomous variables distinguishing males from females.

Educational background, or *education*, is also a similar key component to the analyses. Education was measured as level of education. The respondents were asked "Which is the highest level of education you have achieved." In the case of the Finnish data, the response options were "Primary school," "Vocational school," Secondary school," "College degree," "Degree in applied sciences," or "University degree." In the American questionnaire the response options were "Less than a high school diploma," "High school diploma," "Some college," "A college degree," or "A master's degree, professional degree or higher." For both the Finnish and American data, the level of education is used as dichotomous variable throughout the book, separating those with at least a college degree from those with less education.

Modern societies have heterogeneous populations. Racial background, ethnicity and immigration status are important factors contributing to varying life orientations and life chances. Our survey included a question on immigration status. We simply asked, "Were you born in the United States/Finland," with response options being "yes" and "no." In addition, the American samples also included a question on respondent's race. We relied on standard racial categories that have been developed by the American Census Bureau. The categories of this measure included: "White," "Black or African American," "American Indian or Alaska Native," "Asian," and "Native Hawaiian or Other Pacific Islander," as well as "Hispanic or Latino." The questionnaires also offered an option for individuals who identify with more than one race, namely "Two or more races." In our analyses, we use information on race as a dichotomous measure, categories being "white" and "other" because of the relatively small number of respondents identifying as some of the racial categories. Moreover, race was not asked in Finland because of European Union conventions. Given that Finland's population is approximately 1% Black, race becomes a near-constant in the Finnish data. We therefore only use race as a dichotomous variable.

Many of the chapters use information on respondent's *political preference*, or political affiliation. With this information, we can compare those who support

## 186 *Methodological Appendix*

the political regime in power against those who support political opposition. Our questionnaires included a question: "Which of the following political parties is most important to you?" The question included a list of the party affiliations in the country. The Finnish questionnaire included several options since Finland is a multi-party country. The options were: "Social Democratic Party," "Center Party," "Green League," Left Alliance," "Swedish People's Party," "The Finns Party," "Coalition," "Christian Democrats," and "Movement Now." In addition, there was an option for those who preferred not to say. American questionnaire included four options: "Democrat," "Republican," "Independent," and "Prefer not the say."

In Finland, the situation in 2020 was that the Government consisted of five parties: "Social Democratic Party," "Centre Party," "Green League," "Left Alliance," and "Swedish People's Party." Preferences for these parties were labeled as "Government party supporter," and the remaining ones as "Other." In the American sample, the party preference variable is dichotomized between "Republican" and "Other" as the United States government was led by a Republican at the time of the original 2020 surveys. Table AI gives descriptive statistics (means or percentages) for all background variables by country and survey round for 2020 data.

Table AI

|  | USA R1 | USA R2 | FINLAND R1 | FINLAND R2 |
|---|---|---|---|---|
| Age (mean) | 48.8 | 45.7 | 46.5 | 45.4 |
| Age group | | | | |
| 16–24 (%) | 12.7 | 14.3 | 11.3 | 12.8 |
| 25–34 (%) | 17.0 | 16.0 | 15.5 | 15.1 |
| 35–44 (%) | 17.8 | 18.5 | 18.3 | 18.4 |
| 45–54 (%) | 19.3 | 18.2 | 19.8 | 19.2 |
| 55–76 (%) | 33.3 | 32.9 | 35.1 | 34.4 |
| Sex | | | | |
| Female (%) | 53.6 | 53.0 | 52.5 | 52.3 |
| Education | | | | |
| At least college (%) | 57.2 | 51.5 | 46.8 | 47.0 |
| Immigration status | | | | |
| Born outside country (%) | 8.7 | 8.4 | 3.5 | 4.1 |
| Race | | | | |
| White | 76.5% | 74.5% | – | – |
| Political preference | | | | |
| Supports party in power (%) | 32.5 | 31.5 | 36.1 | 35.7 |
| Panel respondent | – | 39.9% | – | 48.8% |

*Methodological Appendix* **187**

## Specific Measures

The following describe variables that were used in the chapters. For the demographic variables described above, the reader is directed to "see background variables." The operationalizations of other concepts are provided below. Several concepts were used in multiple chapters, but we only include the operationalization of those variables in the initial chapter in which they appear. Subsequent chapters refer the reader to the chapter where the variable's operationalization is described.

### *Chapter 1*

No empirical analyses were conducted in the introductory chapter. The data that were used are secondary data and the sources of these are described in the chapter.

### *Chapter 2*

Variables used in this chapter include:

- *Age* (see background variables).
- *College degree* (see background variables).
- *Country* (see background variables).
- *Perceived causes of the pandemic.* This concept was measured using the item, "In your opinion, what contributed to the coronavirus outbreak becoming a pandemic?" Respondents were asked about 12 possible contributors, and they indicated if they strongly disagreed, disagreed, neither disagreed nor agreed, agreed, or strongly agreed with each contributor. The 12 possible contributors were:
  o Wildlife street markets.
  o Ineffective politics.
  o Leisure travel.
  o Weak restrictions.
  o Business travel.
  o Global overpopulation.
  o Internet fake news.
  o Lack of responsibility.
  o Loose morals.
  o Immigrants.
  o Global economy.
  o Climate change.
- *Planned behavioral changes.* These were measured with the question: Please, tell us how likely you will do each of the following in future? Respondents were asked about 11 possible behavioral changes, and they were asked to indicate if the change was "not at all applicable," "somewhat applicable," or "applicable" for each behavior. The behaviors included:
  o I will make online purchases more often than earlier.
  o I will order food to home more often than earlier.

**188** *Methodological Appendix*

- I will buy takeout food more often than earlier.
- I will avoid public gatherings.
- I will use public transport less than earlier.
- I will visit bars and restaurants less often than earlier.
- I will generally travel less than earlier.
- I will fly less often than earlier.
- I will visit friends and relatives less often than earlier.
- I will use programs like Zoom, Skype, Facetime or other computer tools for interpersonal communication more often than earlier.
- I will purchase online services (e.g., movies, exercise) more than earlier.
- *Planned changes to interactions* and *planned changes to consuming behaviors.* The above planned behavioral change items were factor analyzed to create these two concepts. The first reflected planned changes to interactions with the questions about avoiding public gatherings, using public transportation less, traveling less, flying less, visit bars and restaurants less often, and visit friends and relatives less often. The second factor reflected planned changes to consuming behaviors with the questions concerning using computer programs like Zoom and FaceTime more, purchasing online services more, making online purchases more, order food for home more often, and ordering take-out food more often. The two-factor solution accounted for 64.37% of the variance in the 11 items, and the commonalities ranged from 0.513 to 0.733 (Table AII).

The factor loadings were:

Table AII

| | Component | |
| --- | --- | --- |
| | **Interactions** | **Consuming Behaviors** |
| Avoid public gatherings | 0.725 | 0.284 |
| Use public transport less | 0.688 | 0.297 |
| Visit bars and restaurants less often | 0.756 | 0.279 |
| Generally travel less | 0.808 | 0.297 |
| Fly less often | 0.748 | 0.309 |
| Visit friends and relatives less often | 0.716 | 0.353 |
| Use programs like Zoom more often | 0.388 | 0.602 |
| Make online purchases more often | 0.429 | 0.668 |
| Order food to home more often | 0.208 | 0.809 |
| Buy take-out food more often | 0.210 | 0.796 |
| Purchase online services more | 0.343 | 0.748 |

*Methodological Appendix* **189**

- *Sex* (see background variables).
- *Worry about COVID-19.* The extent to which respondents were worried above COVID-19 was measured with the item, "How worried are you about the coronavirus pandemic? Responses were "not at all," "slightly," and "very much."

## Chapter 3

Variables used in this chapter include:

- *Age* (see background variables).
- *College degree* (see background variables).
- *Country* (see background variables).
- *Perceived causes of the pandemic* (see Chapter 2 variables).
- *Political preference/party in power* (see background variables).
- *Sex* (see background variables).

## Chapter 4

Variables used in this chapter include:

- *Age* (see background variables).
- *College degree* (see background variables).
- *Country* (see background variables).
- *Confidence in central institutions and confidence in press; and confidence in science.* We measure confidence in institutions the same way as in our previous paper (Sedgwick et al., 2022). It was measure using a factor analysis of items asking respondents if they had a great deal of confidence, only some confidence, or hardly any confidence in the people running 12 major institutions including: banks and financial institutions, major companies, organized religion, the executive branch of the federal government, the legislative branch of the federal government, the legal system, the media, the press, the scientific community, education institutions, and medicine or healthcare. The general stability of the factor solutions was apparent in the loadings with three dimensions emerging in both nations: *confidence in central institutions* (banks, major companies, organized, religion, executive branch, legislative branch, the legal system, organized labor), *confidence in the press* (Press, media), and *confidence in science* (scientific community, education, medicine, or healthcare). Only confidence in science was used in this chapter, but the factor scores for all three dimensions are presented in Table AIII.

## 190 *Methodological Appendix*

Table AIII

|  | Factor 1 | Factor 2 | Factor 3 |
| --- | --- | --- | --- |
| Banks | **0.671** | 0.222 | 0.159 |
| Major companies | **0.671** | 0.275 | 0.088 |
| Organized religion | **0.673** | 0.158 | 0.013 |
| Executive branch | **0.741** | 0.071 | 0.094 |
| Legislative branch | **0.538** | 0.434 | 0.123 |
| Legal system | **0.477** | 0.310 | 0.338 |
| Military | **0.577** | −0.133 | 0.422 |
| Organized labor | **0.404** | **0.491** | 0.206 |
| Press | 0.146 | **0.844** | 0.166 |
| Media | 0.179 | **0.846** | 0.126 |
| Scientific community | 0.082 | 0.193 | **0.784** |
| Education | 0.167 | 0.251 | **0.661** |
| Medicine | 0.082 | 0.193 | **0.784** |

- *Feelings of isolation*. Respondents were asked "How often do you feel isolated from others?" The response categories were hardly ever, some of the time, and often.
- *Future prospects*. To measure the respondents' future prospects, they were asked to rate "your prospects for the future" on an 11-point scale ranging from (0) very bad to (10) very good.
- *Life satisfaction*. Respondents were asked how they would rate "You satisfaction with your life" on a scale from 0 (very unsatisfied) to 10 (very satisfied).
- *National debt*. Respondents were asked to state if they strongly agreed, agreed, were neutral, disagreed, or strongly disagreed with the statement, "It is acceptable for the USA/Finland to take on more national debt because of the pandemic."
- *Perceived causes of the pandemic* (see Chapter 2 variables).
- *Political preference/party in power* (see background variables).
- *Race* (see background variables).
- *Sex* (see background variables).
- *Sick due to COVID-19*. Respondents were asked, "Have you or a family member suspected to become sick due to the Coronavirus." The responses were no (coded as 0) and yes (coded as 1).
- *Spending priorities*. To measure respondents' spending priorities, they were provided with the following prompt: "Some argue that government spending needs to change because of COVID-19. In your opinion what should happen to public spending on the following areas?" The responses were (1) cuts can be made, (2) current public spending needs to be maintained, or (3) requires additional public spending. Factor analysis to identify three

*Methodological Appendix* **191**

areas: *welfare, development,* and *security.* "Welfare" spending includes funding allocated to (a) the public sector, (b) public healthcare, (c) public schools, (d) pensions, (e) social benefits, (f) scientific research, and (g) universities. "Development" spending includes funding to support (a) development aid, (b) immigration costs, (c) culture and the arts, (d) environmental protection, (e) support of business, and (f) transportation infrastructure. "Security" spending category is comprised of (a) military and (b) police. The three-factor solution accounted for 48.4% of the total variance (Table AIV). The following factor scores were obtained for each dimension.

Table AIV

|  | **Factor 1** | **Factor 2** | **Factor 3** |
|---|---|---|---|
| Public sector | **0.439** | 0.433 | 0.102 |
| Public healthcare | **0.788** | 0.003 | 0.086 |
| Public schools | **0.601** | 0.2520. | 0.114 |
| Pensions | **0.534** | 0.021 | 0.335 |
| Social benefits | **0.625** | 0.268 | −0.014 |
| Scientific research | **0.609** | 0.152 | 0.085 |
| Universities | **0.491** | 0.405 | 0.106 |
| Development aid | 0.191 | **0.739** | 0.047 |
| Immigration costs | 0.024 | **0.786** | 0.042 |
| Culture and arts | 0.155 | **0.695** | 0.080 |
| Environmental protection | 0.425 | **0.538** | −0.056 |
| Support business | 0.168 | **0.357** | 0.332 |
| Transport infrastructure | 0.197 | **0.422** | 0.334 |
| Military | −0.056 | 0.230 | **0.787** |
| Police | 0.240 | −0.129 | **0.770** |

- *Social capital.* The measure of social capital is a composite measure of five, five-point Likert items. Respondents were asked if they strongly agreed, agreed, neither agreed or disagreed, disagreed, or strongly disagreed with the following statements:
  o I am proud to be a member my community.
  o I feel I am part of my community.
  o People in my community share the same values.
  o I trust my neighbors.
  o People work together to get things done for this community.

## 192 *Methodological Appendix*

These were combined into an index with alphas of 0.864 in Finland, 0.871 in the United States, and 0.864 on the combined samples.

- *Total media consumption.* Respondents were asked about the following media consumption behaviors:
  - o Watch television.
  - o Listen to radio.
  - o Read print media in the form of news or periodicals.
  - o Follow political or societal news in traditional media (e.g., television, newspapers, radio).
  - o Use the Internet.
  - o Read online news or periodicals.
  - o Listen to radio programs or podcasts online.

Responses were coded as 0 news sources, 1 news source, 2 news sources, and 3 or more news sources.

- *Worry about COVID-19* (see Chapter 2 variables).

### Chapter 5

Variables used in Chapter 5 include:

- *Age* (see background variables).
- *College degree* (see background variables).
- *Country* (see background variables).
- *Daily media consumption.* This concept refers to the number of different media platforms used daily by respondents in the month prior to being surveyed. Respondents were asked, "During the past month, how often did you ..." Their usage was reported on a scale from 1 to 10 ("Not once." "Once," "More than once but not weekly," "Once a week," "Several times a week," "Once a day," "Several times a day," "Once an hour," "Several times an hour," and "All the time"). Respondents were asked about the following media consumption behaviors:
  - o Watch television.
  - o Listen to radio.
  - o Read print media in the form of news or periodicals.
  - o Follow political or societal news in traditional media (e.g., television, newspapers, radio).
  - o Use the Internet.
  - o Read online news or periodicals.
  - o Listen to radio programs or podcasts online.

These platforms were categorized into three types: (1) broadcast media, such as television and radio; (2) journalistic media, including newspapers and magazines; and (3) social media, encompassing social networking sites and discussion forums. To focus on the daily consumption patterns, a binary variable was created

*Methodological Appendix* **193**

grouping "not once" through "several times a week" into one category (coded as 0) and "once a day" or more frequently into another category (coded as 1).

- *Satisfaction with the government's handling of the crisis.* Respondents were asked "How satisfied are you with the government's handling of the COVID-19 crisis?" They reported their level of satisfaction on a scale from 1 to 10, with 1 being not satisfied and 10 being very satisfied.
- *Trust in experts.* Respondents were asked, "How likely do you think each of the following groups or institutions will contribute to ending the COVID-19 pandemic?" The responses were "none at all," "a little," "some," and "a lot." The groups or institutions asked about were "university researchers," "doctors or medical experts," and "epidemiologists." These were combined into a summative index to measure *trust in experts.*
- *Sex* (see background variables).

### Chapter 6

The following variables were used in Chapter 6:

- *Age* (see background variables).
- *College degree* (see background variables).
- *Country* (see background variables).
- *Exposure to online hate.* Respondents were asked: "During the past 3 months, have you seen hateful or degrading writing or speech online inappropriately attacking individuals or groups?" Responses were yes and no.
- *Online news consumption* (see Chapter 4 variables).
- *Sex* (see background variables).

### Chapter 7

Variables used in this chapter include:

- *Age* (see background variables).
- *College degree* (see background variables).
- *Country* (see background variables).
- *Coping strategies.* Respondents were told they would be asked about items that "deal with ways you've been coping with the stress in your life since the start of the COVID-19 pandemic." They were then asked, "Which of the following apply to you personally?" The coping strategies asked about included the following:
  - o I've been turning to work or other activities to take my mind off things.
  - o I've been concentrating my efforts on doing something about the situation I'm in.
  - o I've been saying to myself "this isn't real."
  - o I've been using alcohol or other drugs to make myself feel better.
  - o I've been getting emotional support from others.

## 194  *Methodological Appendix*

o   I've been giving up trying to deal with it.
o   I've been taking action to try to make the situation better.
o   I've been refusing to believe that it has happened.
o   I've been saying things to let my unpleasant feelings escape.
o   I've been getting help and advice from other people.
o   I've been using alcohol or other drugs to help me get through it.
o   I've been trying to see it in a different light, to make it seem more positive.
o   I've been criticizing myself.
o   I've been trying to come up with a strategy about what to do.
o   I've been getting comfort and understanding from someone.
o   I've been giving up the attempt to cope.
o   I've been looking for something good in what is happening.
o   I've been making jokes about it.
o   I've been doing something to think about it less, such as going to movies, watching TV, reading, daydreaming, sleeping, or shopping.
o   I've been accepting the reality of the fact that it has happened.
o   I've been expressing my negative feelings.
o   I've been trying to find comfort in my religion or spiritual beliefs.
o   I've been trying to get advice or help from other people about what to do.
o   I've been learning to live with it.
o   I've been thinking hard about what steps to take.
o   I've been blaming myself for things that happened.
o   I've been praying or meditating.

These items were factor analyzed. The four-factor solution accounted for 54.4% of the total variance in the 27 items. Communalities ranged from 0.398 to 0.784 (Table AV). The factor loadings were:

Table AV

|  | Factor 1 | Factor 2 | Factor 3 | Factor 4 |
| --- | --- | --- | --- | --- |
| Getting over with alcohol or drugs | **0.781** | 0.018 | 0.174 | 0.000 |
| Refusing to believe it's real | **0.706** | 0.230 | −0.133 | 0.239 |
| Repeating it's not real | **0.632** | 0.246 | −0.089 | 0.247 |
| Feeling better with alcohol | **0.782** | 0.017 | 0.172 | −0.023 |
| Self-criticizing | **0.647** | 0.338 | −0.034 | 0.061 |
| Giving up dealing with it | **0.657** | 0.248 | −0.068 | 0.147 |
| Giving up coping | **0.717** | 0.221 | −0.064 | 0.169 |
| Joking | **0.470** | 0.191 | 0.308 | −0.161 |
| Blaming self | **0.734** | 0.201 | −0.066 | 0.221 |
| Repeating for escaping feelings | **0.466** | 0.491 | 0.059 | 0.134 |
| Getting emotional support | 0.172 | **0.740** | 0.123 | 0.095 |

Methodological Appendix    **195**

Table AV    (*Continued*)

|  | Factor 1 | Factor 2 | Factor 3 | Factor 4 |
|---|---|---|---|---|
| Getting comfort and understanding | 0.168 | **0.729** | 0.151 | 0.098 |
| Turning to work | 0.130 | **0.487** | 0.350 | 0.126 |
| Getting help and advice | 0.235 | **0.740** | 0.081 | 0.072 |
| Altering current situation | 0.113 | **0.487** | 0.350 | 0.126 |
| Coming up with action strategy | 0.115 | **0.489** | 0.352 | 0.279 |
| Getting advice what to do | 0.354 | **0.683** | 0.038 | 0.160 |
| Doing to think less | 0.135 | **0.454** | 0.273 | 0.126 |
| Thinking next steps | 0.162 | **0.529** | 0.285 | 0.234 |
| Expressing negative feelings | 0.414 | **0.499** | 0.064 | −0.082 |
| Thinking more positive | 0.159 | 0.378 | **0.451** | 0.263 |
| Making situation better | 0.036 | 0.411 | **0.435** | 0.397 |
| Accepting the reality | −0.156 | 0.172 | **0.713** | −0.097 |
| Learning to live with it | −0.081 | 0.065 | **0.745** | −0.014 |
| Looking for good sides | 0.103 | 0.270 | **0.535** | 0.335 |
| Religion or spirituality | 0.216 | 0.177 | 0.037 | **0.835** |
| Praying or meditating | 0.168 | 0.181 | 0.082 | **0.847** |

The analysis resulted in the following four coping styles: *Factor 1* (maladaptive coping): Repeating it's not real, Feeling better with alcohol, giving up dealing with it, refusing to believe it's real, getting over with alcohol and drugs, giving up coping, joking, blaming self, self-criticizing. *Factor 2* (active/expressive and planning coping): Turning to work, altering current situation, getting emotional support, saying unpleasant feelings, getting help and advice, coming up with an action strategy, getting comfort and understanding, doing to think less, expressing negative feelings, getting advice what to do, thinking about next steps. *Factor 3* (positive reframing): Making situation better, thinking more positive, Looking for good side, Accepting the reality, Learning to live with it. *Factor 4* (religious coping): Religion or spirituality, praying or meditating.

- *Life satisfaction* (see Chapter 4 variables).
- *Married*. Respondents were asked about their living situation. Those who were married or living with a partner were considered to be "married" (coded as 1), while those who were living alone, a single parent, living with parents, or living in some other family type such as living with a roommate were considered to be "not married" (coded as 0).
- *Self-esteem*. Respondents were asked how they would rate "Your self-esteem" on a scale from 0 (very unsatisfied) to 10 (very satisfied).

## 196    Methodological Appendix

- *Sex* (see background variables).
- *Social capital* (see Chapter 4 variables).
- *Worry about COVID-19* (see Chapter 2 variables).
- Confidence in Science (see Chapter 4 variables).

### Chapter 8

Variables used in this chapter include:

- *Age* (see background variables).
- *College degree* (see background variables).
- *Collaborative dimensions.* Collaborative dimensions refer to the extent to which respondents view the relationship between themselves and their state as a collaborative partnership. There are five collaborative dimensions (Sedgwick et al., 2022): (1) governance, (2) administration, (3) norms of trust, (4) mutuality, and (5) autonomy. All of the questions measuring these dimensions were ordinal and have response categories of (a) not at all applicable, (b) somewhat applicable, (c) applicable, and (d) very applicable. The items included the following:
  1. I understand my role in preventing the spread of COVID-19.
  2. I can find information easily about how to prevent the spread of COVID-19.
  3. The COVID-19 health (prevention) guidelines are clear for me to follow.
  4. If everyone follows the guidelines for how to reduce the spread of COVID-19, we will be able to combat the pandemic.
  5. I follow the guidelines to protect myself or my family.
  6. I follow the guidelines to protect my community.
  7. It is challenging to follow the COVID-19 health guidelines.

  Administration is measured by item 1, governance includes items 2 and 3, norms of Trust are measured with item 4, mutuality is measured items 5 and 6, and autonomy is measured with item 7.

- *Confidence* in science (see Chapter 4 variables).
- *Country* (see background variables).
- *Married* (see Chapter 7 variables).
- *Mask wearing.* The concept was measured with the item, "I wear a mask when in public." The response categories were (a) not at all applicable, (b) somewhat applicable, (c) applicable, and (d) very applicable.
- *Political preference/party in power* (see background variables).
- *Sex* (see background variables).
- *Social capital* (see Chapter 4 variables).
- *Vaccine intention.* The concept was measured with the item, "I will get a COVID-19 vaccination if one is developed and shown to be safe." The response categories were (a) not at all applicable, (b) somewhat applicable, (c) applicable, and (d) very applicable.
- *Worry about COVID-19* (see Chapter 2 variables).

## Chapter 9

Because this chapter uses the third wave of data, the operationalizations of the variables used in this chapter are described in the chapter.

## Chapter 10

No additional empirical analyses are conducted in the final chapter.

# References

Dynata. (2024). *Tap into Dynata's proprietary 70 million consumers and business professionals.* https://www.dynata.com/generate-new-data/

Parti, K., Dearden, T., & Hawdon, J. (2025). Perspectives of paid panel survey research in cybercrime victimization and offending: Validity of global online market research sampling and data collection. In R. Graham, S. Humer, C. Lee, & V. Nagy (Eds.), *Routledge international handbook of online deviance* (Chapter 6). Routledge.

Sedgwick, D., Hawdon, J., Räsänen, P., & Koivula, A. (2022). The role of collaboration in complying with COVID-19 health protective behaviors: A cross-national study. *Administration & Society, 54*(1), 29–56.

Simmons, A., & Bobo, L. (2015). Can non-full-probability internet surveys yield useful data? A comparison with full-probability face-to-face surveys in the domain of race and social inequality attitudes. *Sociological Methodology, 45*(1), 357–387.

Weinberg, J., Freese, J., & McElhattan, D. (2014). Comparing data characteristics and results of an online factorial survey between a population-based and a crowdsource-recruited sample. *Sociological Science, 1,* 292–310.

# Index

Ability, Benevolence and integrity model (ABI model), 68
Accounting for cross-national differences in exposure to hate during pandemic, 95–96
Acts of terrorism, 30
Adaptive coping strategies, 110, 116–118
Age, 40, 95
American data, 41
American respondents, 22
American welfare model, 8
Analytic technique, 35–36
Anti-statism, 9
Anti–Asian hate, 99–100
Attitudes, 17, 33
Attrition analysis, 72

Behaviors (changed due to COVID-19), 5
Binary logistic regression model, 95
Black Lives Matter movement (2020), 57
BRIEF Cope, 111
Broadcast media, 72
Business, 58

Center for Disease Control (CDC), 4, 156, 177
Central Intelligence Agency (CIA), 7
CEOWORLD Magazine's Health Care Index, 7
Changes to consuming behaviors, 15, 22, 188
Changes to interactions, 15, 22, 188
Chinese government, The, 98
Climate change, 175
Collaboration theory, 152
Collaborative dimensions, 196

Collaborative relationship, 153, 159
Comparative analysis, factors affecting, 134–138
Comparative data analyses, 184
Compliance, importance of health–protective behaviors and, 127–128
Compliance with health mandates, 162
Computer programs, 23
Confidence, 53, 172, 175–176
confidence/trust in science, 57
in experts, 161–162
in institutions, 157, 162
Consistent messaging, 176
Consuming behaviors, 23, 25
Contact tracing, 152
and testing, 148–149
Coping
analyzing predictors of coping strategies, 111–117
anticipate findings, 110
anticipated findings, 118–120
factors affect, 109–110
on life satisfaction, 120
relationship between quality of life and, 117
strategies, 11, 108
Coronavirus (COVID–19), 4–6, 16, 30, 36, 43, 97–98, 113
COVID-19-related deaths, 145
cross-national context of, 18–20, 50
data, variables, and analytic technique, 35–36
descriptive analysis, 36–38
differences in public perceptions, 34–35
Finland and United States, 7–10
impact on American and Finnish Societies, 6–7, 10–12

## 200 Index

importance of online hate during, 88–89
interpretations on evolution of COVID-19 pandemic, 31–34
online hate during COVID-19 pandemic in Finland and United States, 91–94
outbreak, 66
outcomes, 146
pandemic, 31, 53, 57, 71, 86, 108, 127, 133, 144, 160, 177, 180
predicted perceptions of causes of pandemic in United States and Finland, 47
predictive analysis, 38–41
symbolic interactionism and, 129–134
Counter-messaging, 178
Crisis
  management, 66
  media, 70
  trust during, 175–180
  trust in experts during, 67–69
Cross-national approach, 6
Cross-national context of COVID-19, 18–20, 50
Cross-national differences, 10–11, 22, 25
  accounting for cross-national differences in exposure to hate during pandemic, 95–96
  and implications, 162–163
  logistic regression of exposure to online hate in Finland and United States, 95
Cyberbullying, 87
Cyberstalking, 87
Cyberviolence, 87

Daily media consumption, 72
Data, 35–36
  collection procedure and description of variables, 183–184

Debt-to-GDP ratio, 51
Democratic Biden administration, 153
Democrats, 129
Demographic variables, 187
Development, 55
Digital services, 34
Digital technologies, 33
Discussion forums, 68
Disease severity, 19
Dynata company, 183

Early perceptions, COVID-19, 145–146
Education, 39, 185
Education level, 72
Educational background, 185
Effective messaging in a crisis/crisis messaging, 116
Emergency Powers Act (Finland), 32
Emotion-oriented coping, 120
Emotional-based coping mechanism, 114
European Social Survey, 23
Experts, media use and trust in, 70–71
Expressive and Planning Coping, 111

Face coverings, 149–150
Facebook, 87
FaceTime, 23
Factor loading scores, 111
Fairness Doctrine, The, 173–174
Fake News/Reports, 33, 38
Fear, 86
Federal Bureau of Investigation (FBI), 88
Filter bubbles, 88, 173
Finland
  COVID-19, 7–10
  Criminal Code, 90
  landscape of online hate in, 89–91
  online hate during COVID-19 Pandemic in, 91–94
Finnish law, 164
Finnish residents, 112, 115, 134, 137
Finnish respondents, 23, 57, 91
Freedom of speech, 7

## Index    201

General background variables,
    measurement and
    description of, 184
Gini coefficient, 9
Global phenomena, 33
Government, 69
    funding allocated in response to
        pandemic, 52
    parties, 40
Government Stringency Index, 150
Governmental agencies, 156

Hate crimes, 88–89
Hate speech, 90, 99
Health outcomes, COVID-19, 146
Health recommendations and health
    outcomes, COVID-19,
    146–152
Health-protective behaviors, 126,
    164
    importance of health–protective
        behaviors and compliance,
        127–128
    mean compliance and difference
        with mask wearing in
        Finland and United
        States, 127
Health-protective behaviors, typical
    factors affect compliance
    with, 128–129
Healthcare system, 156
Human-caused disasters, 30

Immigration, 24, 38, 41–42
Indirect coping mechanism, 114
Influenza Pandemic, The (1918), 4
Inglehart–Welzel's secularism, 7
Institutional system, 69
Institutional theories of trust, 70
Institutions, 53
    spending vital and confidence in
        institutions necessary for
        public support, 56–59
Inter-relatedness of collaborative
    dimensions, 157
Interactions, 24

International Monetary Fund (IMF),
    50
International movement, 32
International Telecommunication
    Union (ITU), 7
Internet, 34, 178
Interpersonal resources, 110
Ivermectin, 145

John Hopkins University CSSE
    COVID-19 Data, 18
Journalistic media, 72

Klu Klux Klan (organized hate
    groups), 87

Landscape of online hate in Finland
    and United States, 89–91
Law enforcement, 57
Life satisfaction, 49, 117, 119–120,
    160
Lockdowns, 148
Logistic regression analyses, 152
Long-term consequences, COVID-19,
    145–146

Maladaptive coping, 117–118
Maladaptive strategies, 160
Married/marital status, 195
Mask wearing, 126, 128, 133, 145,
    152
Masks, 6, 33, 132
Mass shootings, 30
Media, 173
    consumption, 67, 71, 75
    environments, 67
    use and trust in experts, 70–71
Medical community, 156
Mental health, 108
Middle East respiratory syndrome
    (MERS), 16
MERS-CoV, 4
Mitigation strategies, 18
Multi-national studies, 91
Multilevel analysis, 75
Multivariate analysis, 53

## 202  Index

National debt, willingness to
increasing, 50–51
Negative indirect coping strategy, 109
Next crisis, trust before, 172–175
Non-medicinal health preventative
measures, 126

ODIHR, 89
Omnivorous media consumption, 153
Online hate
during COVID-19 pandemic,
88–89
during COVID-19 pandemic in
Finland and United States,
91–94
exposure, political rhetoric, and
policy implications, 99–100
importance of, 86–88
landscape of online hate in
Finland and United States,
89–91
materials, 91
Online personalizing algorithms, 173
Online services/eCommerce, 23
Organized hate groups, 87

Pandemic, 79, 126
accounting for cross-national
differences in exposure to
hate during, 95–96
causes of, 24
contact tracing and testing,
148–149
cross-national differences and
implications, 162–163
early perceptions and long-term
consequences, 145–146
face coverings, 149–150
government funding allocated in
response to, 52
health recommendations and
health outcomes, 146
mitigation efforts, 148
peek back, 160
planned behavioral changes for
dealing with, 21–22

regression of collaborative
relationship with State in
United States and Finland,
158
restrictions and shutdowns,
150–152
results, 154–156
state as collaborative partner,
157–159
vaccination prediction, 152–153
vaccines, 146–148
Perceived behavioral control, 17
Personal protective equipment (PPE),
4, 174
Planned behavioral changes to
mitigate COVID-19's
effects
changing interactions vs.
changing consumer
behaviors, 22–24
cross-national context of
COVID-19, 18–20
planned behavioral changes for
dealing with pandemic,
21–22
planned changes and beliefs about
pandemic's causes, 24–26
TPB, 17–18
Polarization, 26, 100
Political affiliation, 35
Political divides, 172–173
Political party, 130, 154
affiliation, 159
in power, 53
Political preferences, 38, 42
Political trust, 66
Positive indirect coping strategy, 109
Positive reframing coping, 111, 114,
116
Pre-recruited panel surveys, 184
Predictive analysis, 38–41
predicted perceptions of causes of
pandemic in Finland, 40
predicted perceptions of causes
of pandemic in United
States, 39

President Trump
  anti-mask rhetoric, 133
  COVID-19 rhetoric and effect on
    hate, 96–99
Press freedom, 9
Primary explanatory variables, 77
Prime Minister Marin's COVID-19
    rhetoric and effect on hate,
    96–99
Principal Components Analysis
    (PCA), 22n3
Print media, 79
Public debate, 31
Public health officials, 127
Public priorities during pandemic
  cross-national context of
    COVID-19, 50
  factors predicting public spending
    priorities in Finland and
    United States, 54
  government funding allocated in
    response to pandemic, 52
  spending vital and confidence in
    institutions necessary for
    public support, 56–59
  support for welfare, development,
    and security spending,
    53–56
  willingness to increasing national
    debt, 50–51
Public spending, 50, 52
Public support, spending vital and
    confidence in institutions
    necessary for, 56–59
Public trust in institutions, 56

Quality of life
  anticipated findings, 118–120
  relationship between coping
    strategies and, 117

Rally effect, 69
Random-effect within–between
    models (REWB), 74
Raw material supply arrangements, 33
Regression analysis, 38, 113, 119, 137

Religion, 90, 115
Religious coping, 117–118
Republican Party, 42
Resilient communities, 162
Respondents, 55
Risk perceptions, 43
Risk society, 30

Scholars, 128
Science, 5, 53
Secularism, 7
Severe acute respiratory
    syndrome coronavirus 1
    (SARS-CoV-1), 16
Severe acute respiratory syndrome
    coronavirus 2
    (SARS-CoV-2), 4, 16, 33
Sex/gender, 40, 185
Shutdowns, 152
Sickness (Covid-19), 8–9, 146
Skepticism, 179
Social capital, 53, 57, 110, 112, 191
Social connectedness, 110
Social context, 17–18
Social distancing, 126, 145, 152
Social media, 68, 72, 88
Social networking
    platforms, 87
    sites, 68
Social networks, 129
Social norms, 17
Social pressures, 128
Social relationships, 110
Social response to COVID-19
    pandemic, 31
Social science, 5
Sociological literature, 30
Solidarity, 157
Spanish Flu, 4
Spending, 52–53
Spending on defense, 55
Spending on welfare, 53, 55, 57
Spending vital and confidence
    in institutions necessary
    for public support,
    56–59

## 204 Index

State as collaborative partner, 157–159
Statist, 172
Stringency index, 150$n$3
Survey data, 5, 10
Symbolic interactionism
and COVID-19 pandemic, 129–134
factors affect compliance with mask wearing, 131
Symbolic interactionist approach, 129

Television, 79
Theory of Planned Behavior, 11
Theory of Reasoned Action, 17
TPB, 17–18
Trade, 33
Traditional journalistic print media consumption, 78
Traditional news media platforms, 79
Trust, 136, 161, 172, 176
analysis procedure, 74
during crisis, 175–180
in experts and government success, 69–70
in experts during crisis, 67–69
in institutions, 126, 128–129
literature review, 67
measures, 72–74
media use and trust in experts, 70–71
before next crisis, 172–175
participants, 72
results, 74–79
in social relations, 66

TTSC, 108
framework, 121
research, 110
Twitter, 87

United States (US)
Center for Disease Control, 108
COVID-19, 7–10
government, 176
landscape of online hate in Finland and, 89–91
online hate during COVID-19 pandemic in Finland and, 91–94
residents, 115, 134
respondents, 53

Vaccines/vacination, 146–148
factors affecting vaccine uptake, 134–138
prediction, 152–153
Variables, 35–36
Voluntary compliance, 68

Welfare spending, 52
Welfare state, 8
Welfare systems, 9
Well-being, 108, 117–118, 146, 160
White House Coronavirus Task Force, 145
World Health Organization (WHO), 4, 98, 108, 179
Worry about Covid, 53, 116, 130

Zoom, 23

Printed and bound by CPI Group (UK) Ltd, Croydon, CR0 4YY
05/02/2025

14638644-0001